CW00573311

Published in Australia by
Iridium Press
Perth, Western Australia

Disclaimer: The material in this publication is of a general nature, and should be used as a guideline only. Readers should obtain professional advice where appropriate, before making any such decision. To the maximum extent permitted by the law, the contributors, authors and publishers disclaim all responsibilities and liability to any person, arising directly or indirectly from any person taking or not taking action based upon the information in this publication.

National Library of Australia Catologuing-in-Publication entry
Author: Meek, Julie
Title: Truth, Lies & Chocolate: 99 Facts and Fairytales About Food
ISBN: 978-0-9806767-0-9
Category: 1 Nutrition 2 Performance 3 Well Being

Second Printing 2010

Editor: Jo-Anne Craine, Type A Creative
Illustrations: Natalee Poli
Cover & Book Design: Madhouse Design
Printed: Geon Advance Press

This book is printed on Monza Satin Recycled paper

BLEACHING PROCESS   MANAGEMENT SYSTEMS   FOREST MANAGEMENT   RECYCLED CONTENT

truth, lies & chocolate

99 Facts and Fairytales About Food

Julie Meek

IRIDIUM PRESS

For my Aunty Rona, who taught me...
"There is no such thing as can't."

Foreword

There are lots of books about food and nutrition. As an Accredited Practising Dietitian, I've read my fair share of them, and I'm amazed at the quantity of misinformation out there.

As a certified specialist in my field, I've spent my life helping clients sort through mountains of nutrition half-truths and propaganda. Over the years I've gathered a stack of the most common facts and fallacies; and now I've assembled 99 of them to provide you with the truth.

Every day I help my clients find the simple solution to their health questions as good eating habits plus the right food choices equals good health. This book reflects the many questions, myths and mistakes people make about nutrition. I know it can help you too.

Feel free to flip through these pages any way you like. Theres no need to read it from cover to cover; it's designed to let you graze and nibble at information that you can easily digest at your own pace. Open it to any page and discover the answers to popular misconceptions and you'll learn some new facts you can apply to make healthier changes to your life instantly.

Happy reading, but more importantly happy eating!
Julie Meek, Accredited Practising Dietitian

1. Is chocolate good for you?

"I never met a chocolate I didn't like." - Deanna Troi in Star Trek: The Next Generation

Cocoa and chocolate products are made from cacao (Theobroma cacao) beans and it has become evident that they are a rich source of antioxidant flavonoids.

Chocolate lovers will be happy to know that there is increasing evidence from clinical and experimental studies showing favourable health effects of chocolate. These benefits may include: an increase in antioxidant activity and reductions in blood pressure, inflammation, LDL cholesterol, and an overall reduction in cardiovascular risk. (Hooray!)

Such studies have shown that cocoa and chocolate contain a high quality and quantity of antioxidant flavonoids, exceeding other well known sources such as black and green tea and red wine. But before you grab your favourite candy bar, note that this is only primarily true of dark chocolate, which contains 2-3 times as many cocoa flavonoids as milk chocolate. However, keep in mind that the flavonoid content of dark chocolate is dependent on the percentage of cocoa used and the manufacturing process, which can destroy flavonoids.

At this point in time, although experts know that dark chocolate has some very positive health effects; there is not enough evidence to form the basis of a public health recommendation for daily intake.

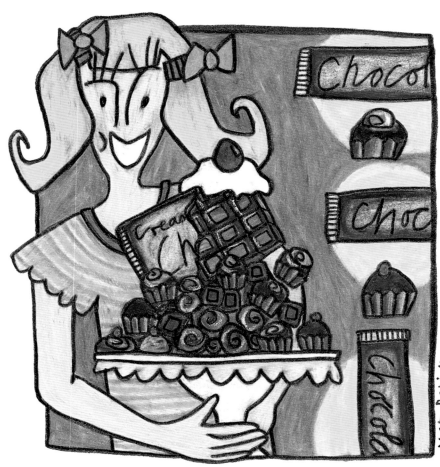

Chocolate is famous, the international rock star of sweets. Let's face it, when Katherine Hepburn talks about you, you have made it.

There are books, poems, movies, and websites dedicated to it. The Swiss take the gold medal for consuming the most chocolate in the world, at 10-12 kg per capita annually. Australia ranks a lowly 11th in the world for wolfing down chocolate, according to the Association of Chocolate Biscuits and Confectionary Industries (2005).

The world's largest manufacturer of chocolate, Barry Callebaut, has released a product called Acticoa that contains 80% of the flavonoids found in raw cocoa. This cocoa can be used in chocolate drinks, desserts, biscuits, confectionery fillings and snacks. Other companies including Hershey's are jumping on the bandwagon and have released antioxidant milk chocolate and Whole Bean Chocolate® items onto the market.

We need to be mindful that chocolate is relatively high in calories and fat. However, if you are eating a healthy, balanced diet and leading a healthy lifestyle, it is important that you indulge in food that you love, including a little chocolate now and then.

"What you see before you, my friend, is the result of a lifetime of chocolate."
- Katherine Hepburn

2. Is decaffeinated coffee harmful to your health?

When decaffeination of coffee first began in 1903, benzene was the solvent used. Due to health concerns it is no longer used in the process. The solvents used today have to pass regular testing and stringent criteria, so you can drink decaf coffee without worrying that it is harmful to your health.

For those of you that love coffee, 'decaf' may be a dirty word. You may be surprised to know that decaffeinated coffee accounts for 10% of the coffee market globally.

Decaffeination is the act of removing caffeine from coffee beans, cocoa, tea leaves and other caffeine-containing materials. To be classified as decaf, coffee must be 97% free of caffeine.

Coffee is quite a complex substance and contains over 400 chemicals that are important to its taste and aroma. There is no physical process or chemical reaction that will remove only caffeine while leaving the other chemicals at their original concentrations. Coffee beans are decaffeinated in their green bean form before roasting and the process occurs by a few different methods. Recently, a coffee Arabica bean naturally low in caffeine was found in Ethiopia and perhaps this could replace chemically treated coffee in the near future. Potentially, genetic engineering could also create a 'naturally caffeine-free' coffee.

3. Does tea contain as much caffeine as coffee?

The amount of caffeine in your cup of tea will depend on how you make your tea and how long you let it brew (or steep). Generally speaking, one cup of tea will contain only half to one third as much of the caffeine in one cup of coffee. Many people mistakenly believe that green tea is completely caffeine-free. It's not. Caffeine-free or low caffeine tea is available at supermarkets, but be aware they still do contain trace amounts of caffeine. The following table shows a comparison of some commonly consumed beverages and their caffeine content.

Tea is the world's second favourite drink (Water is first). There are three principal categories; black, green and oolong, which originate from the same plant, Camellia sinensis. Herbal teas are not technically teas but infusions of plants or herbs and are naturally caffeine-free.

Caffeine Counter		Caffeine (mg)
Brewed Coffee	1 cup	85-120
Instant Coffee	1 cup	60
Brewed Tea	1 cup	75
Instant Tea	1 cup	30-50
Green Tea	1 cup	50-80
Decaf Tea	1 cup	2
Cocoa Powder	2 tsp	20
Energy Drink	250ml	80
Milo	2 tsp	1
Cold Drinks	375ml	40
Herbal Tea	1 cup	nil

4. Is coffee a good source of antioxidants?

Unproven. It has been known for some time that fruit and vegetables, tea, dark chocolate and red wine are all rich sources of antioxidants. Coffee has been lurking in the background and it would now seem that it has something much more to offer than just a boost of energy to get us going for the day.

'Antioxidants' is now a buzzword in the field of nutrition and although much research is ongoing, they may be of great benefit in tackling modern health problems such as cancer, heart disease, eye disease and the unavoidable issue of aging.

Coffee contains a particular type of antioxidant called chlorogenic acid (a combination of caffeic and quinic acid) and this is likely to represent the majority of coffee antioxidants. Roasting coffee beans increases their total antioxidant activity, and the antioxidant content of coffee is comparable to other beverages such as tea and red wine.

Some research has shown that drinking 3-4 cups of coffee per day can reduce the risk of developing certain chronic diseases including Type 2 diabetes and dementia. The mechanisms behind this are not yet fully understood and further research is needed to clarify these findings.

This research is emerging and certainly potentially exciting for coffee lovers!

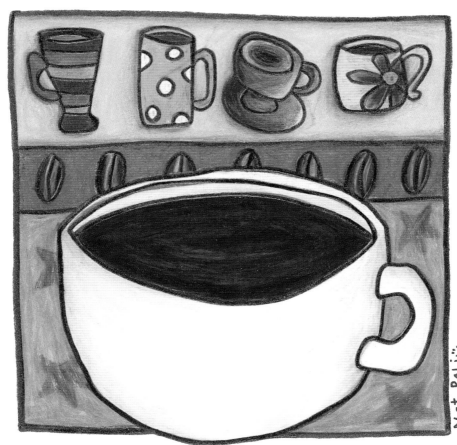

Nat Polic.

5. Is the combination of calories, or total calories, more important in a daily diet?

Both, actually. It does matter what your total calorie or kilojoule intake is derived from - and it is not advisable to use them all up on your favourite snack of Mars Bars® or Tim Tams®! All calories are not treated equally. When considering weight loss there is a simple, irrefutable fact. Many people like to gloss over this bit. What goes in (food) must be less than what goes out (exercise).

Calories are derived from fat, alcohol, protein and carbohydrate and this is where we get our food energy. Calories or kilojoules are essentially the petrol to run our 'car' - the human body.

Our energy requirements are highly individual and dependent on factors like age, activity level, weight and height. It is true that the body does not treat the above nutrients equally.

Food Energy	Energy per gram
Nutrient	
Fat	37 kJ (9 kcal)
Alcohol	29 kJ (7 kcal)
Protein	17 kJ (4 kcal)
Carbohydrate	16 kJ (4 kcal)

If alcohol has been consumed, it is your body's first choice as a fuel source. This means that it is used as petrol by your body first, in preference to fat, protein and carbohydrate. If fat is also being consumed at the same time, (perhaps in the form of nuts and chips at the pub on a Friday night after work!) then the fat consumed will be diverted into fat storage even more efficiently! Bad news.

Carbohydrate and protein calories that are in excess of our needs are used for energy, and displace fat yet again as an energy source. This means that they are the second priority for energy use. Carbohydrate is stored in the muscle and liver and the capacity for storage is quite low, whereas protein stores are mainly in the muscle and their size is dependent on need. Carbohydrate and protein are the main regulators of appetite and produce the feeling of 'being full'. This leaves fat as the last choice for fuel and it has the greatest storage capacity. So remember that fatty food will stick around a long time!

While this order of fuel usage may be true for many people, there will be some people who burn their fuel in a completely different way.

When you lower your total daily energy intake (kJ or kcal) the greater your need to ensure you obtain enough of other nutrients such as zinc, iron, Vitamin B12, omega-3 fatty acids and calcium which are vitally important to your daily diet.

Many popular weight loss diets contain 5500-6000 kJ (1800 kcal) and at this level, the carbohydrate content has to be lower to enable other nutrient needs to be met. It is also important in lower calorie diets to ensure that the carbohydrate based foods are predominantly low glycemic index and should include vegetables, wholegrain cereals, legumes and fruits to maximise nutritional balance.

6. Do children grow out of 'puppy fat'?

Not always. Obese children in Australia have a 25 to 50% chance of becoming obese adults. Their chances are increased even further if their parents are overweight or obese and if the child remains overweight as a teenager. Research shows that the risk sits around 80% if both parents are overweight or obese and 40% with one parent being overweight. Being obese or overweight can cause many problems, not just the physical variety. It can result in emotional and social health problems too.

The statistics on obesity in Australia are not looking good. The rate of overweight children doubled, and childhood obesity tripled in Australia between 1985 and 1995. Studies in Australia indicate that around 30% of girls and boys are currently overweight or obese and it does seem that this is an increasing trend in particular parts of our population. There are many factors involved in Australia's weight problems at all levels of society; but encouraging healthy eating and exercise is the best way to prevent obesity.

As a parent, it is your responsibility to help your child find ways to stay active and be one of the 70% of kids in the healthy range. Don't dismiss the significant weight issues of your older child as just puppy fat. An active, healthy child has a greater chance of growing into an active, healthy adult.

7. Are higher protein diets effective for weight loss?

Protein heavy diets like "The Atkins Diet" have become popular internationally. The ability of higher protein diets to affect weight loss has been assessed in several scientific studies in Australia and overseas. In Australia in 2003 the effectiveness of a higher protein, low fat diet was evaluated in a study with 100 overweight or obese women. It was found that the group who were eating the most protein lost the most weight, and additionally, lost more weight specifically around the abdomen than the other test group. From this study, the CSIRO Total Wellbeing Diet was born.

Protein plays several roles in weight loss. It helps you feel fuller for longer and therefore reduces total food and calorie intake. Higher proportions of protein and lower proportions of high glycemic index carbohydrates may aid people with Type 2 diabetes or metabolic syndrome. Another point to consider is that in low calorie diets, a higher protein intake is essential if nutrient needs are to be met. Protein foods are major sources of iron, zinc, vitamin B12, calcium and long-chain omega-3 fatty acids. However, you must be sure not to eliminate other healthy foods like fruits and vegetables for the sake of a higher protein diet.

A diet with plenty of protein derived from foods such as red meat would not be the first choice for a vegetarian, therefore higher protein diets are not for everyone.

If you are unsure about which path to take, professional judgment is always advisable. Accredited Practising Dietitians have the knowledge and skills to help you decide the best avenue to take, as there is now a choice of effective, clinically proven approaches to weight loss.

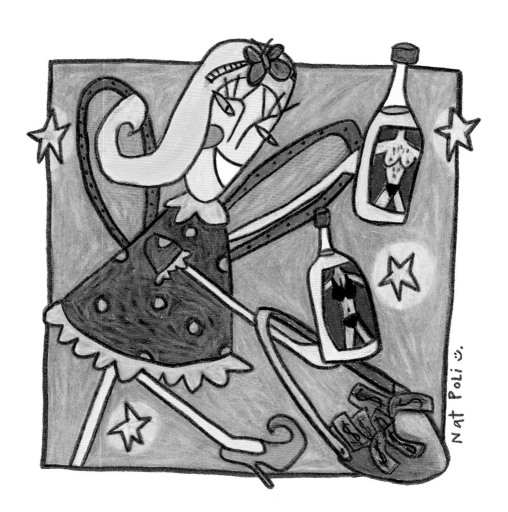

Nat Poli

8. Is it possible to pick a gimmick or fad diet?

Pick up any magazine and you will find a reference to a 'diet' in there somewhere. The term 'diet' is very negative and makes people do all sorts of bizarre things (like eating a block of chocolate instead of one piece) and generally makes them unpleasant people to be with. The expression "going on a diet" implies that one day you will come off the diet. Healthy eating is about changing your habits and enjoying food, not making your life a misery.

Given that there are many wonder diets out there in fantasyland, how can we pick one that works? You may find the following checklist helpful.

- ☐ Does it claim to have 'magic' ingredients e.g. grapefruit, seaweed or vinegar?
- ☐ Does it promise rapid weight loss - like the diet that guarantees a loss of 13 inches around one leg?
- ☐ Do you have to exercise or do you just have to lie on a vibrating machine that 'shakes' the fat off?
- ☐ Who is selling the program - are they qualified and do they hold a recognised degree in nutrition or does it seem like the 'diet' is a quick way for them to make some cash?
- ☐ Do you have to buy expensive powders, potions, pills or creams that claim to miraculously melt away fat?
- ☐ Are you guaranteed weight loss in specific areas of your body?
- ☐ Do you have to eat a small range of foods that are not familiar to you and perhaps you have never heard of before?
- ☐ Does the diet teach you new and improved eating habits or is it a crash course in how to count calories?

We need to be savvy when considering changing our eating habits. If you discover what seems to be a promising eating plan, run it through the checklist. It highlights all the features of the fad diet that you should avoid. Seek professional advice from an Accredited Practising Dietitian if you would like specific information on what encompasses a healthy diet.

9. Are nuts fattening?

This depends on the volume of nuts you consume. Many people love to sit down with a bowl of nuts for a snack. But is it a healthy option? Yes – in small portions. Nuts do contain quite a lot of fat and are therefore high in kilojoules. You should take this into consideration if you are watching your weight, and choose the raw, unsalted varieties. The table below shows the fibre, fat and kilojoule content of some common nuts.

Research shows that nuts are very nutritious and contain mostly polyunsaturated and monounsaturated fats, which we know are good for our hearts and cholesterol levels. They are also a good source of protein, fibre, Vitamin E, magnesium and selenium.

Type of Nut	Fibre (g)	Fat (g)	Kilojoules (kJ)
Per 1/2 cup measure			
Almond	7.5	46.5	2065
Cashew	4.5	37	1795
Macadamia	4.5	55.5	2210
Peanut	6.5	36.5	1800
Walnut	3.5	38	1570

There is also emerging evidence to suggest that an increase in nut consumption may reduce the risk of developing Type 2 diabetes. This is great news considering it is estimated 1 million Australians have diabetes and half don't know they have it. (Diabetes WA)

Most people would find it relatively easy to eat ½ cup of nuts and this would provide around one quarter of the total daily kilojoule intake for most women and some men.

The Australian Guide to Healthy Eating recommends a handful (30 grams) of nuts five times weekly for good health.

10. Does grapefruit burn fat stores faster?

No. You may have heard that grapefruit and other citrus have magical properties to assist weight loss and fat burning. That would be lovely, but unfortunately there is no food or herb that causes miraculous weight loss and the two key factors for losing weight are diet and exercise. There are many fad diets around and the Grapefruit Diet is one of them. This diet originated in South Africa in the 1960s as a means of clearing a seasonal grapefruit glut. Grapefruit and other citrus fruit are good sources of fibre and Vitamin C and should be included as part of a regular diet, but they do not have special components that aid weight loss.

11. I'm getting married, am I going to turn into a blimp?

Congratulations! There are some studies which show that being married is associated with improved health overall. However, there have been few studies conducted internationally on the issue of weight gain and marriage and there is a perception amongst some that once married; the weight piles on.

The clinical studies that have examined weight in relation to marital status have produced various debatable results. More consistent results come from studies which report some weight gain early in marriage, and in an Australian study that followed couples for 2-3 years after marriage, husbands (but not wives!) gained weight. Men and marriage have also been associated with weight gain in longer term studies. Could this be because newly married men are happily enjoying proper home cooking?

In a West Australian study involving 39 couples in Perth, researchers found evidence suggesting that weight gain and a decrease in physical activity emerge as problems early in the period of adjustment for couples beginning their lives together. Another group of researchers in the United States found that in the 9043 adults they studied, entering or leaving marriage did influence physical characteristics such as body weight, both gained and lost.

Ultimately, you are the master of your own destiny and this is also true of your health behaviour after marriage. If you work together to maintain healthy eating patterns and get your bodies moving, serious weight gain will not be a concern.

12. Does eating too much sugar cause diabetes?

No. Although eating too much sugar can cause a variety of health issues, it does not cause diabetes.

It is estimated that about 1 million people in Australia have diabetes and half of them don't know they have it! Type 1 (insulin dependent) diabetes is an autoimmune condition. Autoimmune conditions occur when the body's immune system is triggered and the normal function of organs becomes abnormal, in this case the pancreas. In Type 1 diabetes, a gene triggers the immune system and the gene is thought to be stimulated by a viral infection. This infection may damage the pancreas beyond repair, resulting in complete insulin deficiency.

With Type 2 diabetes, insulin production may not be working properly and can result in eventual exhaustion of the pancreas. This is the most common type of diabetes. It is not known what causes Type 2 diabetes but the risk factors are thought to be family history, lack of physical activity, excessive body fat and aging.

13. Should I eat carbohydrate after 5pm?

I often get asked if it is okay to eat carbohydrates after 5pm when clients are trying to lose weight and I usually ask a question in return. Does your body know what time it is? There is nothing magical about this time, it has been chosen randomly and is not based on fact.

There is not one single scientific study that lends support to the theory that carbohydrates need to be cut out after 5pm. In addition, no recognised health authority endorses this theory either. While it doesn't make sense to eliminate carbohydrate foods at the evening meal, if you usually have large portions at dinner, then reducing the amount you eat could be advisable. Type 2 diabetics are one group of people who should definitely not cut out carbohydrates after 5pm as this could cause their blood sugar levels to drop too low.

If you want to lose weight, try these suggestions instead:

- Reduce the total amount of food that you eat - it will have a greater impact than cutting out carbohydrates.
- Eating more vegetables can also help reduce the amount of other foods on your plate.
- Eating earlier in the evening gives your body a chance to use up some of that meal's food energy before bedtime.
- Try an after-dinner walk to burn off a few extra calories and stimulate your metabolism.

Remember that carbohydrates are often not the sole source of weight gain. Extras like cream sauces, cheese and other added fats (e.g. butter on bread) are often the real culprits.

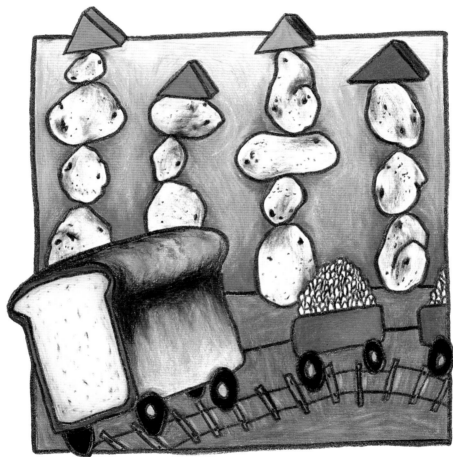

14. Are all carbohydrates created equal?

No. Carbohydrates used to be classified as simple or complex based on the speed of digestion. This type of classification assumed that 'simple' carbohydrates (lollies, soft drink, cordial, honey, etc.) were digested quickly and 'complex' carbohydrates (breads, cereal, rice and pasta, fruit and vegetables) were digested slowly. Research has progressed significantly and we know that there is more to it than digestion speed. As carbohydrate foods are digested and absorbed, the blood glucose level rises and this promotes the release of insulin. Insulin promotes the storage of glucose into cells and lowers blood sugar levels.

Research has shown that a carbohydrate food can be classified according to how quickly it is digested and more importantly, how quickly it is absorbed into the bloodstream as glucose. This classification is known as the Glycemic Index (GI). Simply stated - low GI foods are digested and absorbed slowly and high GI foods quickly.

When carbohydrates are tested, the food under scrutiny is eaten and their effects on blood glucose levels are measured. All foods are compared to 50g of glucose, which has a GI of 100. A GI of 60 means that a carbohydrate-containing food raises blood sugar levels to 60% of pure glucose. Since a meal you eat may contain several carbohydrates the GI of a meal is approximately the average of the GI foods in the meal. Many other aspects of a meal can affect the overall GI including fat, fibre, protein, cooking methods and food preparation.

The GI of some foods may surprise you. Rice Bubbles® have a higher GI than cordial. Multi-grain bread has a higher GI than white chocolate.

This doesn't really change our nutrition advice. If you eat minimally processed and higher fibre foods such as fruits and vegetables and wholegrain cereals with minimal 'treats', your diet is likely to be mostly low GI. This is because they are not easily converted to glucose and take longer to be absorbed. Carbohydrates with higher fibre content tend to be more filling, allowing you to better control your appetite and body fat.

15. Is raw or brown sugar better for you than white sugar?

No. It is often thought that raw or brown sugar is the 'wholemeal' variety of sugar. However, all sugar is 100% carbohydrate and provides kilojoules or calories but little else. Apart from flavour, there is no advantage in replacing raw and brown sugar or honey for white sugar. One teaspoon of sugar contains 80 kilojoules, which is equal to two jellybeans. Consider that when you are next about to spoon sugar into your coffee.

The average Australian consumes 45 kg of sugar per year.

16. Should proteins and carbohydrates be combined in the same meal?

Yes. The human body is very clever and does not get confused about the particular job that it is doing at any given time. So when some carbohydrates and protein come sailing down the intestinal tract, the digestive juices in the small intestine supply the correct enzymes to complete the job of digesting carbohydrates to sugars, proteins to amino acids and fats to fatty acids. And, because the human body is multi-skilled, all of these processes happen at the same time.

This theory of food combining is based on the 1985 "Fit for Life" book. This is a diet based on the assumption that carbohydrates such as pasta, rice, bread, potato and cereals should not be eaten at the same time as proteins; which includes foods such as dairy products, meat, chicken, fish, eggs and nuts. The meal plan suggests one fruit meal per day (usually breakfast), one protein meal per day and one carbohydrate meal per day. Many foods we eat contain both carbohydrates and proteins in the same item.

In practical terms this means that if you were having spaghetti bolognaise for dinner, you need to eat the meat sauce at lunchtime and the spaghetti at dinnertime! This type of meal plan is neither realistic nor enjoyable.

People have lost weight on this diet, but not because they avoided carbohydrates and proteins in the same meal. It is more than likely due to them eating less food overall and choosing more nutritious foods.

17. Is sugar addiction a genuine disease?

No. Although there is no genuine disease related to 'sugar addiction', you may feel a strong craving for sugar and sugary foods. Eating these foods may have become a habit and you may feel a compulsion to continue eating them. The Dorland's Medical Dictionary defines addiction as "physiologic or psychologic dependence on some agent with a tendency to increase its use." Sugar is pretty much 100% carbohydrate and would not be classified as an 'agent' in any context.

Having said that, when we eat foods that are high in carbohydrates and low in protein, our brains release a neurotransmitter called serotonin, which makes us feel happy. Serotonin influences the control of our mood and behaviour.

Moods can be affected when blood sugar levels fluctuate more, as they do when carbohydrates with a high glycemic index are consumed regularly. Carbohydrates that have a low to medium glycemic index provide longer lasting energy and help you feel fuller for longer. Fewer energy dips mean fewer mood swings. And remember, just because you have a craving, it doesn't mean that you have to act on it.

18. Why do I feel very full immediately following a rice-based meal and then hungry again a few hours later?

You have just eaten a rice-based meal and your stomach is full. You wonder whether you will be able to ever eat again because you feel like you might burst and then before you know it, you are hungry again. How can that be? Many of us can relate to this scenario.

Rice is rich in carbohydrate, an excellent source of energy and is a filling and satisfying food. However, the rice you have eaten may have a high Glycemic Index. Being a carbohydrate, rice can be classified by the Glycemic Index. The Glycemic Index of rice varies considerably depending on the brand, colour and cooking method. Some examples are below:

Good choices for more satisfying rice are Doongara, Basmati, SunRice® medium grain brown rice in 90 sec (in pouch) or Mahatma® Long Grain. This means that these types of rice will be absorbed into your bloodstream at a slower rate and result in you feeling fuller for longer. Perhaps it may also result in no more midnight snacks for you!

Rice	GI
Jasmine Rice	109
Calrose® brown rice	87
Sunbrown® Quick rice, brown	80
White rice, medium grain	75
SunRice® Medium Grain brown rice in 90sec	59
Basmati rice	58
Doongara rice	56
Mahatma® Long grain white rice	50

Source: Sydney University Glycemic Index Research Service (SUGiRS) 2005

19. Are soy products healthier than dairy products?

In recent years, soy products have received considerable media attention, both good and bad. Soya beans and soy foods are ancient and have been around for centuries, forming an integral part of many Asian countries diets. They have only been popular in western cultures, like Australia, for a few decades.

We know soya beans are high in fibre, low in fat (especially the 'bad' type), rich in vitamins and minerals and an excellent source of protein. Soya beans have twice as much protein as any other legume and are equal to cow's milk in protein quality. There are numerous scientific studies citing health benefits of including soy foods in the diet. These benefits include lowering cholesterol levels, combating certain cancers, managing menopause and preventing osteoporosis. There are natural compounds found in soya beans called phytoestrogens, which are known as isoflavones in soya beans. It is believed that isoflavones are responsible for some of the health benefits associated with eating soy foods.

Several years ago, there was much media hype about soy foods and their effect on breast cancer. It was suggested that isoflavones might stimulate breast cancer cell growth and therefore increase the risk of developing breast cancer. Isoflavones do resemble estrogen (the female sex hormone), but they only have a fraction of the strength of estrogen.

So, the jury is in. While soy isoflavones have some similarities to estrogen, they are not identical in their effects and there is no scientific evidence to suggest that women with breast cancer or those who are at risk of developing breast cancer should avoid soy foods.

In comparison, dairy foods are one of the five core food groups and are excellent sources of:

- Vitamins A, B12 and riboflavin
- Phosphorus, potassium, magnesium and zinc
- Protein and carbohydrate

These nutrients are important for healthy blood, bone, nervous and immune systems, eyesight, muscle and nerve function, healthy skin, energy levels and growth and repair in all parts of your body.

Soy and dairy products do differ in their calcium content. Soya beans do not naturally contain calcium and it is important to choose soy products that are calcium-enriched. We need to consume slightly more soy milk (350ml) to absorb the same amount of calcium from one serving of dairy milk (250ml).

It is always advisable to include a wide variety of foods in your diet. Including both dairy and soy foods is beneficial to your health and well-being.

20. Should children be given low fat dairy foods?

Babies and children under the age of 2 years are continually experiencing rapid brain and body growth. Because they need plenty of energy and vital fat-soluble vitamins for this development, skim and reduced fat milk are not recommended for children under 2 years of age. However, between the ages of 2-5 years it is reasonable to give reduced fat dairy foods as their diets have ideally expanded to include a wide variety of foods. Reduced fat dairy foods actually contain more calcium than their full fat counterparts while the protein content remains the same.

21. Are dairy products the only sources of calcium?

It is true that dairy products are not the only sources of calcium. Calcium can be found in many other foods besides milk, cheese and yoghurt. The question is; are you prepared to eat 45 tablespoons of sesame seeds to obtain the same amount of calcium that you will find in 250 ml of milk?

People often ask me if they can use sesame seeds, green leafy vegetables or nuts as an alternate calcium source to dairy products. The following table gives an indication of the quantities of some common foods that contain the same amount of calcium as 250ml of milk.

Food	Quantity	Food	Quantity
Almonds	120g	Broccoli	1kg
Apples	7.5kg	Eggs, boiled	18
Apricots, dried	430g	Salmon, canned with bones	140g
Baked beans	900g	Sesame seeds	45 tsp
Bread, wholemeal	20 slices	Spinach	600g

The other factor to consider is that the calcium in dairy foods is absorbed more efficiently than from other sources. This means that although you might be feeling REALLY hungry and manage to munch your way through 7.5 kg of apples, you still won't absorb the same amount of calcium found in 1 cup of milk.

Most people will be able to obtain their average daily requirement of calcium by eating three servings of dairy every day. One serving of dairy is equal to:

- 1 glass (250ml) of milk
- 1 tub (200g) of yoghurt
- 2 slices (40g) of cheese

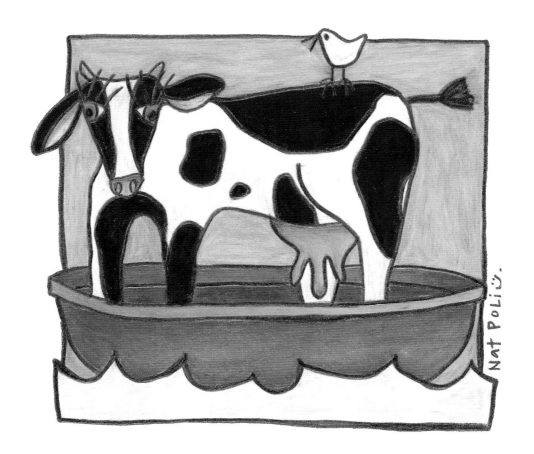

Nat Poli

22. Will eating dairy products cause weight gain?

There is growing scientific evidence that including dairy products in a calorie-controlled diet may actually promote weight loss rather than weight gain. In a recent clinical study it was found that overweight adults on a calorie-controlled diet who included at least 3 servings of dairy foods per day lost 70% more body weight than those on a similar diet with minimal dairy! Studies have shown the same effect on children.

Calcium derived from dairy products appears to influence weight by reducing the amount of fat stored, as well as increasing the amount of fat broken down. Include 3 servings of dairy products per day and you will be on the right path to a healthy weight.

23. Are white spots on fingernails a result of calcium deficiency?

No. White spots or streaks on nails are properly known as leukonychia and are usually caused by injury to the nail bed or plate. Nails can take 8 months to grow out and the spots will disappear accordingly. As your nail grows, the spots will appear to move up the nail over time. There are some real symptoms of calcium deficiency but white spots are not one of them.

24. Can individuals with lactose intolerance consume any dairy products?

Yes. There have been many clinical studies conducted internationally on lactose intolerance and the consumption of dairy products. Nutritionists and a statistician from Purdue University reviewed the studies conducted and found that, based on the evidence currently available, the dose of lactose required to produce symptoms in those with lactose intolerance is approximately 2 cups of milk. Based on this, those who are lactose intolerant could potentially tolerate smaller, single servings of milk (e.g. one cup) throughout the day with meals. This will differ between individuals. Yoghurt and fermented milk products (e.g. Yakult®) are generally well tolerated and hard cheese like cheddar is virtually lactose free. Yoghurt is made from milk using two probiotic species, Lactobacillus bulgaricus and Streptococcus thermophilus, both of which assist in the breakdown of lactose. Lactose-free milk is also available.

Lactose is a sugar found in milk and milk products and when eaten is broken down by an enzyme called lactase. Lactose intolerance is a result of a deficiency in this enzyme and the symptoms of lactose intolerance are abdominal bloating and pain, flatulence and diarrhoea. If milk or dairy food needs to be eliminated it is important to identify alternative sources of calcium. Dairy food is important as our main source of calcium and there is also evidence to suggest that lactose itself assists with the absorption of calcium.

25. When taking calcium supplements, do you need other minerals to aid absorption?

Yes. Vitamin D is essential for increasing the rate of calcium absorption. The cheapest and easiest way of getting your Vitamin D is spending 10 minutes per day in the sun, as this enables the production of Vitamin D within your body. For those people who are unable to do this, such as the institutionalised, and veiled women, a Vitamin D supplement is recommended. Some calcium supplements also contain Vitamin D.

A high salt diet increases the loss of calcium through urine, and therefore it's advisable to minimise the salt content of your diet. There is no evidence to suggest that other minerals such as magnesium have any effect on calcium absorption.

Ideally your calcium intake should be obtained from dietary sources, particularly dairy foods.

Sometimes this is not possible and calcium supplements are required. In the supplement form, calcium is combined with either carbonate or citrate. The two most commonly known calcium supplements are Caltrate (calcium carbonate) and Citrical (calcium citrate). Calcium citrate is more soluble and bioavailable, meaning that it is easier for your body to absorb.

Bone density experts recommend taking calcium supplements in two doses to improve the rate of absorption. The recommended regime is one third of the dose in the morning and two thirds of the dose in the evening.

26. Are fresh fruit and vegetables more nutritious than the frozen and canned varieties?

That depends. Fresh local produce is generally best. Sometimes the quality of frozen fruit and vegetables are superior to fresh if it has to travel far to market, as they can be frozen quickly after being harvested. However frozen food is generally better than canned, as more nutrients are lost in the canning process than for the same food when frozen.

The major nutrient losses that occur in frozen food are not actually related to the freezing process itself but to the blanching that occurs before freezing and then again during cooking. Blanching refers to the process of placing a food into boiling water for a short time and then plunging the food into ice-cold water to halt the cooking process. These losses are not different to those that would occur if you purchase fresh food and cook it at home. Canning involves heating the food in a closed tin, which prevents microorganisms growing and becoming hazardous to our health. The amount of heating depends on the type of food. Nutrient losses occur during heating and storage and some vitamins may dissolve in the liquid in the can.

To make sure that the loss of vitamins and minerals in your fresh and frozen vegetables is kept to a minimum, remember the following:

- Choose fresh fruit and vegetables that are not over-ripe, bruised, cut or scraped
- Avoid peeling unless damaged or unpalatable
- Keep the pieces of food as large as possible when cutting it up

- Add the fruit or vegetables to boiling water rather than to cold water
- Use the smallest amount of water possible, steaming and micro-waving are very effective at minimising nutrient loss
- Cook for the minimum time necessary

27. Should I take a multi-vitamin supplement because vegetables and fruit don't have the same nutritional value that they used to?

Unproven. It is also very difficult if not impossible to determine whether the nutritional value of our fruit and vegetables is less than it used to be, as this type of research was not conducted when vitamins were discovered. Some people believe that our soils are depleted of minerals and as a result our food is lacking in vitamins and minerals. There is no reliable evidence to suggest that this is the case.

Excessive quantities of water-soluble vitamins are mainly excreted in the urine but an excessive intake of the fat-soluble vitamins, A, D, E and K will result in increased storage and potential toxicity.

Billions of dollars are spent each year on nutrition supplements worldwide and there is debate as to whether healthy individuals who eat a well-balanced diet actually require vitamin supplements. This money may be better spent on good quality, healthy food. There are people who may genuinely require vitamin supplementation and they include the elderly, pregnant and breastfeeding women and the chronically ill.

28. Does eating carrots help me see in the dark?

Yes. Carrots are a rich source of beta-carotene, which is a form of Vitamin A. Vitamin A is known as the 'vision vitamin' because it helps prevent night blindness and aids the conversion of light into messages for the brain.

Vitamin A is found in other foods such as butter, margarine, liver, eggs and full-cream dairy products. Green leafy vegetables, yellow vegetables and fruit also contain Vitamin A in the form of beta-carotene.
The daily requirement of Vitamin A is around 750 micrograms and given that ½ cup carrots provides 1087 micrograms, they will definitely help you see in the dark.

Just remember not to get too crazy with carrots. If you overdo the carotene, you can end up with a yellowy, orange colour on your hands and feet. This is probably more of an issue with juicing carrots than eating them.

29. Are avocados fattening?

Avocados do not contain cholesterol but do contain fat, although it is mostly monounsaturated fat, which actually helps lower cholesterol levels. They also contain plant sterols and fibre, which reduce cholesterol absorption in the intestinal tract. If we compare 100g servings of some different types of spreads and their fat content, this is what we find:

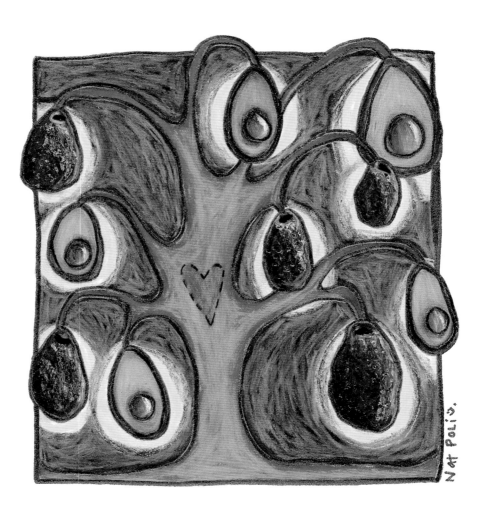

100g Serving of	Amount of Fat
Margarine (any type)	80g
Butter (any type)	82g
Peanut Butter	52g
Avocado	23g

The average serving size of an avocado is considered to be 95 grams or ½ an avocado. This is roughly equal to consuming 1 tablespoon of fat. For a 65kg female who engages in less than one hour of exercise per day the recommended intake of fat is approximately 60 grams. Eating ½ an avocado would provide one-third of her daily fat intake.

So… avocados alone will not cause weight gain and can be a very healthy addition to your diet. Just remember to include them in your daily fat intake.

It might surprise you to know that avocados are known to have existed as far back as 291 BC. The trees originated in the highlands of Central America and Mexico and the lowlands of Colombia in South America. There are actually more than 70 varieties of avocado in Australia. Five of the most popular varieties are Hass, Shepard, Reed, Wurtz and Sharwil.

Avocados are fruit, and they are a well-balanced nutritious package. They contain 14 essential vitamins and minerals and are a good source of Vitamin A, B, C and E, copper, potassium and magnesium. They are also rich in folate, which is essential for prevention of neural tube defects such as spina bifida in unborn babies.

30. Are silver beet and spinach good sources of iron?

When you think of spinach and iron, do you think of Popeye clutching his can of spinach and gulping it down with biceps bulging?

Unfortunately, Popeye did not get his iron and strength from spinach. Dietary iron is found in two forms – haem iron which is found in animal foods and non-haem iron which is found in plant foods. Spinach and silver beet provide non-haem iron, which is not absorbed well by our bodies.

Silver beet is the vegetable with big, dark green leaves and white veins that many people mistakenly call spinach. Silver beet is a close relative of spinach but spinach has a smaller flatter leaf and green veins. Both are good sources of Vitamin A and C, fibre, folate and iron.

Iron deficiency symptoms include tiredness, breathlessness and poor immune function, and this affects one fifth of adult females in developed countries.

31. Is watermelon low in calories/kilojoules due to the high water content?

Yes. Watermelons are 91% water by weight, which means that they are a great source of fluid. They are very good sources of Vitamins A, B and C, potassium, magnesium and the antioxidant lycopene. A 100g serving of watermelon contains 95 kilojoules with a small amount of carbohydrate (5%) and no fat. The same amount of apple contains 205 kilojoules. It makes sense that fruit with higher water content will have fewer calories or kilojoules and this is the case with watermelon.

Some of my best childhood memories are sitting on the back lawn on a hot summer's day with my brother and sisters eating watermelon that my dad had grown; and then having seed-spitting competitions. We ate so much watermelon that I am surprised we didn't start to turn pink!

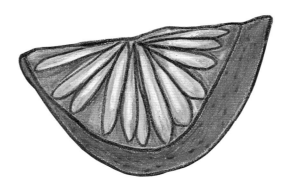

32. Can you eat too much fruit?

It is difficult to consume too much fruit because it is filling and contains quite a lot of water. Fruit is a nutritious and healthy food to include as part of a weight-reducing diet. It is a good source of fibre, although some people can experience diarrhoea or an upset stomach as a result of eating a large amount of fruit. This is more an inconvenience than a health issue.

It is easier to over-eat dried fruit, as it is dehydrated. Six whole dried apricots are equivalent to 6 fresh apricots and a handful of sultanas are the same as eating a bunch of grapes. Tinned fruit can be a good alternative to fresh varieties if the fruit is in natural juice rather than syrup. This reduces the quantity of sugar added to the fruit. Some vitamins will be lost in the canning process (due to heat) but the fibre is retained.

The carbohydrate in fruit is made up mostly of natural sugars, including glucose, fructose and sucrose. The total carbohydrate content varies from approximately 5% in watermelon to 22% in bananas. Most fruits contain between 10-15 percent total carbohydrates, which equates to 10-15 grams of carbohydrate per 100g of the fruit. The Glycemic Index will differ greatly amongst different types of fruit.

Fruit is extremely versatile and can be used as a snack or incorporated into meals and drinks. Many people will be familiar with the Australian government's health campaign which asks us to "go for 2 & 5". This means eating 2 serves of fruit and 5 serves of vegetables per day. Australian adults on average eat 1-2 servings of fruit per day and most should eat more to improve their health. Regularly eating fruit and vegetables can help prevent coronary heart disease, some types of cancer, constipation and obesity.

33. Should diabetics avoid fruit?

The simple answer is no. It is true that fruit does contain sugar as well as fibre but diabetics can tolerate small amounts of sugar without it affecting their blood sugar levels. The fibre in fruit slows down the absorption of sugar into the bloodstream.

Diabetes Australia recommends that diabetics consume at least 2 pieces of fruit daily just like the rest of the Australian population. It is suggested they spread this fruit intake out over the course of the day to avoid blood sugar levels rising too quickly. It is also worthwhile for diabetics to look at the Glycemic Index of various fruit to assess the effect on their blood sugar levels. Have a look at www. glycemicindex.com for the GI of many varieties of fruit. Due to a much higher sugar content and lack of fibre, diabetics are not encouraged to drink fruit juice.

34. Is fruit juice healthy?

When you convert fruit into juice you are left with only the sugar and water and none of the fibre; so it's very easy to drink too much. Fruit juice is not recommended for diabetics and should only be used in very small quantities (or diluted with water) for children. Many people believe that 100% fruit juice is a healthy drink but it still contains sugar. Fruit juice 'drinks' contain a maximum of 50% fruit juice with the remainder being sugar and water.

When you are looking for a thirst quencher pick up the water bottle instead of fruit juice. When buying fruit juice, make sure you choose 100% no added sugar and limit the amount to 1 small glass per day.

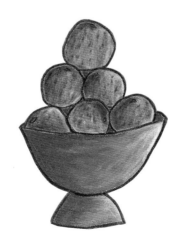

35. Is the colour of vegetables an indicator of their nutritional value?

In part, yes. The colour of vegetables is of much interest in modern day health because nutrition experts know fruit and vegetables are rich sources of antioxidants, and the type of antioxidant they contain is indicated by their colour. Our bodies produce some baddies by the name of 'free radicals' that can cause all sorts of trouble. This is where antioxidants come to the rescue and research has shown that they play a role in cancer, aging, cardiovascular disease and eye disease. Some sources of antioxidants are below:

- Red: good source of lycopene, which helps reduce the risk of prostate cancer in males. Found in tomatoes, watermelon, guava, and ruby grapefruit.
- Orange and Yellow: good source of beta-carotene, which can protect against a range of cancers. Found in pumpkin, sweet potato, carrots, mango, paw-paw, apricots and rockmelon.
- Green: good source of lutein and zeaxanthin, two compounds related to beta-carotene that can protect our eyes as we age. Found in broccoli, spinach, silver beet, capsicum, chilli, parsley and dark lettuces.
- Blue and Purples: good source of anthocyanins for antioxidant and anti-bacterial properties. Found in grapes, blueberries, cranberries, beetroot and radicchio lettuce.
- Brown: good source of catechins for blood vessel health. Found in tea, chocolate and red wine.

Although the 'brown' antioxidants are not related to the colour of vegetables, they are a pleasant surprise!

I remember watching my grandma spoon bicarbonate of soda into her green vegetables while they were cooking and being told that it would keep them nice and green so that they would look good on the plate. Of course, an easier way of doing that is to avoid cooking the living daylights out of them! But it is interesting that there has been curiosity surrounding vegetables and their colour for some time.

So, when you are preparing and choosing your vegetable intake for the day, consider your colour options – eat a rainbow of foods!

36. Does Vitamin C help to prevent colds?

Research has shown that taking large doses of Vitamin C does not prevent you getting a cold but can shorten the duration. Large amounts of Vitamin C (1000mg or 1 gram) can prevent the absorption of other nutrients. Many Vitamin C supplements are at least 250mg in strength, but many people take more than the recommended dose. Fortunately Vitamin C is water-soluble which means that any excess is passed out through the urine, preventing a toxic overdose. The recommended daily intake is 30mg, which is easily achieved by eating fruit and vegetables on a daily basis.

Fruit / Vegetable	Amount	Vitamin C
Kiwi-fruit	1 average	57mg
Orange	1 whole	48mg
Paw Paw	1/3 medium	60mg
Grapefruit	1/2 whole	37mg
Strawberry	12 medium	45mg
Capsicum, Red	1 cup	206mg
Capsicum, Green	1 cup	108mg
Spinach	1 cup	23mg
Broccoli	1/3 cup	43mg
Brussels Sprouts	6	62mg

37. Is canola oil toxic?

No. The canola oil that is available in the supermarket is not toxic. Canola oil is sometimes associated with another oil called rapeseed and it is probably from this connection that the myth has originated. Canola oil is taken from the seed of the canola plant (Brassica napus or Brassica campestris), a variety of rapeseed that belongs to the Brassica family. Although it is derived from the same species of plant, canola oil is different from rapeseed oil in that it has lower levels of erucic acid.

The name 'canola' can only be used if the level of erucic acid is less than 2%. The original rapeseed is only used for non-edible purposes, such as the production of nylon.

38. Is olive oil the best oil to choose for cooking?

Olive oil is only one of a number of healthy oils. It is a monounsaturated fat and others in the same category include canola, peanut, macadamia and avocado oils. All of these oils, in small amounts, are good choices for a healthy heart and do not raise blood cholesterol levels.

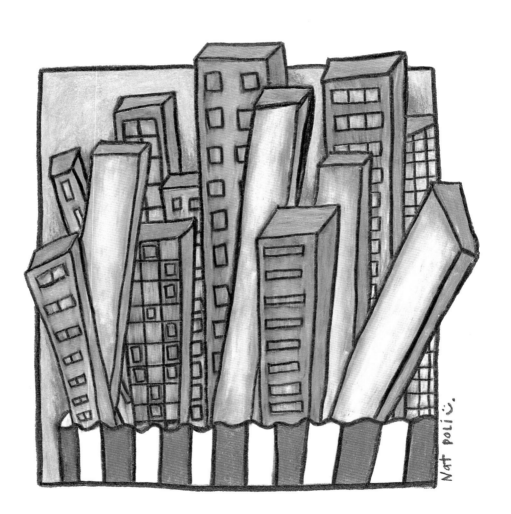

Nat poli☺.

39. Are chips cooked in vegetable oil healthy?

No. Some are better than others depending on what type of oil is being used to fry chips. If your local chip shop cooks their chips in a good quality polyunsaturated or monounsaturated oil, they are a better choice than chips cooked in a saturated fat. However, that's not the end of the story. All varieties of fat, regardless of their type, contain the same quantity of fat per gram. This means that a chip cooked in olive or canola oil has exactly the same amount of fat as a chip cooked in palm oil.

Fats in food are a mixture of three different types known as saturated fat, polyunsaturated fat and monounsaturated fat. The different types of fat have different effects on blood cholesterol levels.

Saturated fat is the type of fat that raises blood cholesterol levels. Since raised blood cholesterol is one of the main risk factors for heart disease, it is a good idea to reduce your intake of foods high in saturated fat. Saturated fat can be found in fatty meat and chicken skin, butter, full fat dairy products, many commercially prepared baked products such as biscuits and pastries and most deep-fried takeaway foods, including chips.

Interestingly, saturated fat is found in two vegetable oils, palm and coconut. These two oils are cheap and commonly used for deep-frying and baking. This means that although takeaway outlets may be advertising that they use vegetable oils, they may not be the healthy variety.

40. Does margarine have fewer calories or kilojoules than butter?

There is no difference in calorie or kilojoule value between margarine and butter. They do contain different types of fat; butter is mainly saturated fat and margarines are mainly polyunsaturated or monounsaturated. Reduced fat spreads are available but make sure you check the label, which will tell you what type of spread you are buying. Be careful not to overuse the 'light' varieties otherwise you will get just as much fat as a scrape of regular margarine.

There are two kinds of fat in everyone's diet. The kind you can see and the kind you can't. You can see the fat in beef, lamb and chicken for instance, but you can't see it in chocolate, pastry, eggs, dairy products and nuts.

What's more, foods like butter and margarine are made entirely of fat. Obviously, it's a lot easier to cut down on the fat you can see. All types of fat have the same calorie level and should be reduced for fat loss.

41. Is butter healthier than margarine?

No. You may see research quoted in the media linking margarine to negative health outcomes. However, this research is not relevant to Australia as it was conducted on US margarines that are often higher in trans fats than Australian margarines. The production of margarine in Australia is different, and many manufacturers have made an effort to reduce trans fat levels. Trans fats are a type of fat found naturally in dairy products, beef, veal, lamb and mutton and may be created during the manufacture of some table margarines, shortenings and solid spreads used in the food industry. It is an unsaturated fat but behaves like a saturated fat in the body and raises blood cholesterol levels.

All margarines with the Heart Foundation Tick have less than 1% trans fats, and these levels are amongst the lowest in the world. On the other hand, butter contains a lot of saturated and trans fat, which raises blood cholesterol levels. High total blood cholesterol is one of the main risk factors for heart disease.

For better health, choose any spread based on canola, olive, sunflower, soybean, safflower, peanut, macadamia, sesame seed and grapeseed oils. Look for margarines that have less than 1% trans fatty acids (check the label) and are low in saturated fat.

42. Do eggs raise blood cholesterol levels?

Research conducted over the past 50 years shows that egg consumption has only a small effect on raising total blood cholesterol levels in healthy people. For most people, eating 3-4 eggs per week is not a major health risk when combined with a low saturated fat diet that includes wholegrain cereals, fruits, vegetables and legumes. It can be an issue if you are frying eggs every day and eating them with lots of bacon and white toast and butter! However, further research is required to fully assess the effects of egg consumption in those people with high cholesterol levels, cardiovascular disease or Type 2 diabetes.

The National Heart Foundation has recognised eggs as a nutritious food with regular eggs eligible for the healthy eating 'Tick of Approval'.

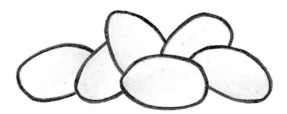

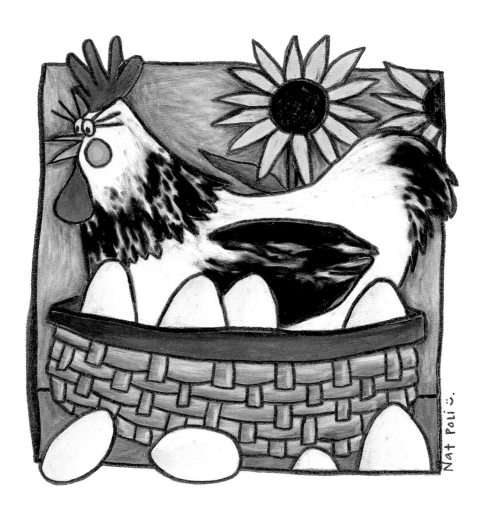

Nat Poli

43. Does cholesterol-free mean fat-free and good for you?

No. Aside from saturated, polyunsaturated and monounsaturated fat there is another type of fat called 'sterols.' Cholesterol is the sterol found in all animal tissues and it can accumulate in the arteries and lead to heart attacks, angina, abnormal heart rhythms and heart failure.

Since cholesterol is only one type of fat, a 'cholesterol-free' product could very well contain other types of fat and is certainly not 'fat-free.'

Ironically, a product claiming to be cholesterol-free could contain saturated fat, which is the type of fat that raises blood cholesterol levels.

44. Are light or 'lite' oils a good way to reduce my fat intake?

No matter how you spell it, light or 'lite' oils have exactly the same quantity of fat and kilojoules as regular oils. In this case, "light" is somewhat deceptive and really means they are only lighter in colour or flavour, and therefore are not lower in fat than regular oils unless they are specifically labelled as such.

45. Can you eat seafood if you have raised cholesterol levels?

You can as long as you use low fat cooking methods such as grilling, bbq and stir-fry; then eating prawns is unlikely to affect your cholesterol levels.

Dietary cholesterol as well as dietary saturated fat elevates blood cholesterol levels. Prawns do contain cholesterol, but they are low in saturated fat and that has a much greater impact on blood cholesterol than cholesterol in food does.

Fish and shellfish, including prawns, are good dietary sources of omega-3 fats and these types of fats play an important role in keeping blood fats at an optimal level and keeping our blood flowing efficiently.

46. Do you get as much omega-3 fats from canned and frozen fish as from fresh fish?

The good news is that canning and freezing fish does not alter the content of omega-3 fats.

Fish, shellfish and fish oils are good dietary sources of omega-3 fats and are found in particularly 'oily' fish such as herring, mackerel, sardines and salmon. Many people don't eat enough fish because they find it too expensive, don't know how to prepare it or find it hard to purchase. This is where using canned or frozen fish can be convenient. To get these great health benefits, eat fish 2-3 times per week; whether fresh, frozen or canned.

Omega-3 fats are fantastic for our bodies. They are multi-purpose and some benefits include:

- Keeping your heart fit and healthy.
- Playing an important role in pregnancy and are especially important for babies' rapidly growing eyes and brains. They also have an integral role in breastfeeding and childhood development.
- Keeping our blood fats (like triglycerides) at optimal levels and keeping our blood flowing freely around our circulatory system.
- Regulating our blood glucose levels, blood pressure and even our heart beat.
- Aiding recovery from coronary heart surgery.
- Boosting brainpower.

47. What are plant sterols in margarine?

Plant sterols or phytosterols are naturally occurring parts of all plant-based food and can be found in vegetable oils, nuts, legumes, fruit, breads, rice and soybeans. Although they are found in food, their concentration is quite low and in recent years this has led to plant sterols being added to some margarines in Australia.

Plant sterols block the body's ability to absorb cholesterol and this reduces the level of cholesterol in the blood. Clinical trials show that a daily intake of 2-3 grams of plant sterols can reduce LDL or 'bad' cholesterol levels by 10% in 3 weeks in most individuals. In practical terms this equates to consuming 1-2 tablespoons of plant sterol enriched margarine every day. It is essential that the full amount is consumed every day to gain the positive effects, as spreading bread lightly with the margarine will have no effect at all.

For those who are concerned with their weight, most of these enriched margarines have a 'light' version that is lower in fat. Decreasing the fat content of the margarine does not affect the concentration of the plant sterols.

Eating plant sterol enriched margarine can be a useful addition to a healthy diet to help lower the concentration of LDL and total cholesterol.

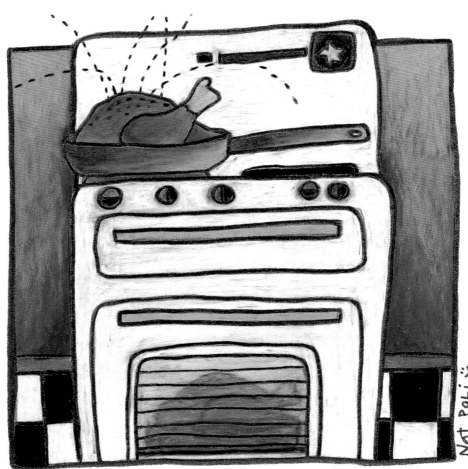

Nat Poli

48. Are food products that are baked rather than fried better for you?

Not necessarily. If food manufacturers bake their products without adding fat it usually is a lower fat product than one that is fried. However, some products are baked with added fat and this results in a very similar fat content to that of fried food. Toasted muesli, for example, is sprayed with oil and then baked, hence 'toasted'.

The most accurate tool is the nutrition label: read it and compare the fat content per 100 grams. For a product to be 'reduced fat' it should contain no more than 8 grams per 100 grams of the product; and 3 grams or less to be 'low fat'.

49. Does frying food damage the nutritional value?

In some foods, yes. The stability of nutrients in food depends on their environment. Nutrients can be lost in food depending on whether the food is exposed to light or air, acid or alkali, the temperature and their ability to dissolve in water.

Frying involves high heat and the greatest nutrient losses affect Vitamins B1 (thiamin) and C. Foods cooked in oil can also have large losses of Vitamin E.

To minimize these losses, cook the food for the least amount of time possible and use only a small amount of oil.

50. Is beer more fattening than wine?

Essentially, standard servings of beer and wine are very similar in terms of kilojoule content and can contribute to weight gain. Beer nutrition. These two words are not usually seen together! Let's do some math. If wine and beer are compared on a 100ml basis this is what we find:

100ml Serving of	Kilojoules
Red Wine	295kJ
White Wine, dry	283kJ
White Wine, sweet	275kJ
Beer, average	149kJ

Fantastic, you think, these figures are reassuring, and beer is looking great. There is a small problem though. Most people don't usually drink just 100ml of beer.

Standard drink servings vary in size depending on the type of alcohol. A standard serving of beer is 250ml or 2/3 can or stubby while a standard serving of wine is 100ml.

Restaurants are more generous when they pour, it seems. An average restaurant size serving of wine is 180ml or 1.8 standard drinks, and the average serving size of a full strength beer is 375ml or 1 middy/can/stubby, which is equal to 1.5 standard drinks.

If you go out and enjoy 2-3 wines or 2-3 stubbys of beer, you will clock up around 1500 -1600 kJ in both cases. This is equivalent to chomping through 4 slices of multi-grain bread, although not quite as nutritious! Beer, wine and other alcoholic drinks can weaken one's resolve and soon have you reaching for high fat snacks. Combining fatty foods with alcohol is the worst combination of all for weight gain, so it is a good idea to eat a meal before drinking alcohol to lessen the temptation to reach for the chips and peanuts.

51. Are low carbohydrate beers the beer equivalent to celery?

Low carb beers are low in carbohydrates but that is not the only source of kilojoules in beer. The average stubby of full strength beer contains 560 kilojoules; light beer contains 360 kilojoules and a low carb beer will contain approximately 470 kilojoules. This means that choosing a low carb beer over a full strength beer will save you about 100 kilojoules.

In a 375ml can or stubby of full strength beer there will be approximately 13 grams of carbohydrate compared to 3 grams in the low carb version. Diabetics may benefit from the lower carbohydrate content but the bigger issue for them is the alcohol content of beer and this is not altered in a low carb beer.

Low carb beers are not new in Australia. The marketing of these drinks is usually accompanied by terms such as 'health and lifestyle conscious', 'low carb diet' and 'for those who like to have a beer but are watching their weight'. Watch out for the false promises of beer advertisers. Low carb beers are not necessarily the same as 'light' beers. Light beers are lower in alcohol.

Drinking low carb beer does not lessen the risks associated with drinking alcohol, such as becoming overweight or obese, cancer, high blood pressure, stroke and birth defects in pregnant women. If you are concerned about your weight, consider choosing a beer that you enjoy and drinking less of it.

52. Is red wine good for you?

It is true that red wine is a rich source of antioxidant flavonols (sub-group of flavonoids). This means that these antioxidants in red wine could lower the risk of cardiovascular disease by reducing the oxidation of LDL cholesterol, the 'baddie' of the bunch and reducing the likelihood of blood clots in our arteries.

The early 1990s were heady days for red wine drinkers. This was when scientists observed that red wine might have some very positive health benefits because it was a good source of antioxidants. Red wine was suddenly celebrated as being good for you at a time when the beneficial quantity was unknown. It meant that there was a perceived license to drink red wine whenever you felt like it.

It is not healthy to drink unlimited red wine and one single glass (100ml) of red wine daily will provide a health benefit. So you can raise your glass for a toast, but don't drink enough to get toasted!

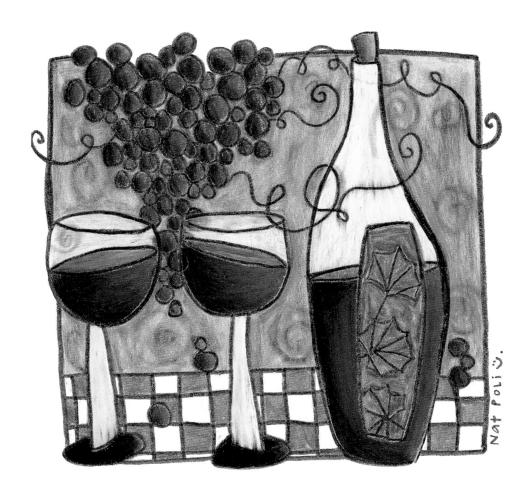

Nat Poli

53. Do you need to eat in the morning before exercising to burn body fat?

Any type of exercise burns body fat, the degree depends on the length and intensity. If you are trying to lose body fat, and your exercise session is not performance driven but rather aimed at fat loss and fitness, then eating after exercise is fine. Remember, it is important not to skip meals because your body needs the energy to exercise. We can't do it on fresh air alone! Some people will find that eating before exercise will give them more energy to perform better, which enables them to burn more kilojoules.

However, if you are an athlete training for or competing in an event, eating prior to exercise will improve your performance. It is advisable to eat 2-3 hours before exercise to allow adequate time for your stomach to empty. This can be difficult if you are training early in the morning and if so, make sure that your meal the night before is high in carbohydrates like rice and pasta. If you can't eat early in the morning try a sports drink or Sustagen® Sport to top up your carbohydrate stores.

The essential thing to know is that any type of exercise burns body fat, and the most important aspect about exercise is that it improves your overall health and reduces your risk of heart disease and other lifestyle diseases. Of course, it also reduces your stress levels and makes you feel good. Just remember to eat breakfast, either before or after your morning workout.

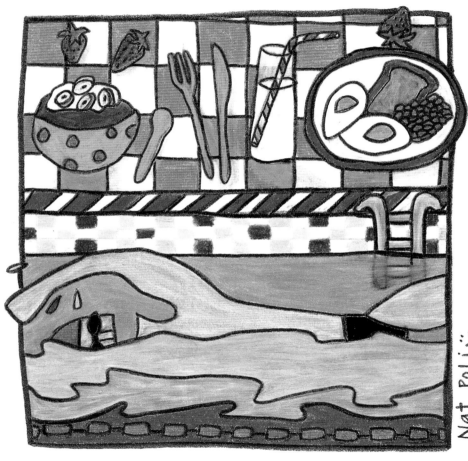

Nat Poli

54. Will protein supplements help build muscles faster?

Not really. Protein supplements won't build your muscles faster than other proteins that are found in food; but consuming adequate protein can certainly assist in muscle growth and repair.

Protein is composed of chains of amino acids and these amino acids are grouped depending on whether they are essential or non-essential. The body can make non-essential amino acids, but not essential amino acids, which can only be provided by food. Essential amino acids can be found in meat, chicken, fish, milk, cheese, yoghurt and eggs. Protein is needed for muscle growth and repair after a resistance type (weight training) training session. The following table demonstrates the protein requirements for various individuals:

Recommended Daily Intake of Protein	
	g / kg (Ideal Body Weight) per day
Adult Australians	0.75
Elite Endurance Athletes	1.6
Endurance Athletes	1.2 - 1.4
Power Sports	1.4 - 1.7
Strength Athletes (early training)	1.5 - 1.7
Strength Athletes (steady state)	1.0 - 1.2
Recreational Athletes	0.9 - 1.2

Athletes do require more protein than the average person, although their concern about consuming adequate protein for peak performance is often more perceived than real. It is not difficult to meet protein needs through food - although there are some athletes who are vegetarian or vegan that may not get enough protein in their diet and may benefit from a protein supplement. This may also apply to professional athletes who have a massive energy requirement and can't achieve this through normal food intake.

Actual Daily Intake of Protein	
	g / kg (Body Weight) per day
Average Australian Adult	1.0 - 1.5
Average Female Athlete	1.0 - 2.8
Average Male Athlete	1.5 - 4.0

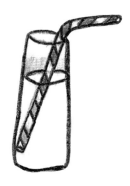

55. Will taking a protein supplement after exercise aid recovery?

According to sports science experts around the world, protein is most important for muscle recovery following exercise. Athletes should aim to consume 10 grams of protein within 1-2 hours following training, and the earlier, the better. Luckily, protein is found in many common foods that we eat, so generally, protein supplements are not required. Some examples of foods containing 10 grams of protein include a peanut butter sandwich, a handful of trail mix (fruit and nuts), an energy bar, a 200g tub of yoghurt or a glass of Sustagen®.

Much controversy surrounds the use of protein supplements. Protein supplements are mostly used by athletes and it seems that often marketing is ahead of science with regards to their use. The nutrition supplement industry is massive, and accounts for billions of dollars spent annually.

Protein accounts for only 3-5 % of the energy produced during exercise, and there is no scientific evidence that indicates consuming protein during exercise is beneficial to performance.

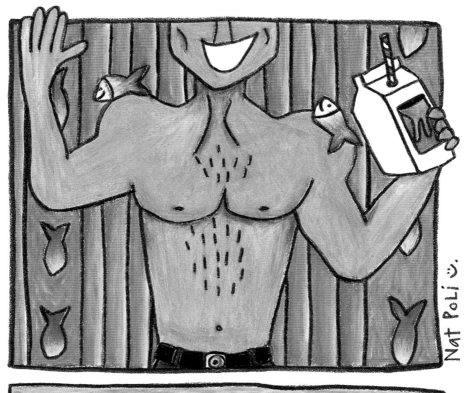
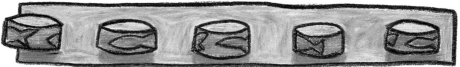

Nat Poli ☺.

56. Are protein powders good value for money in comparison to food?

No. Protein powders appear to be used quite widely within the fitness industry despite the fact that they contain modest amounts of protein at a high cost. These supplements are usually in a powder form that can be added to or made into a drink. They are a mix of two or more ingredients including: milk protein, egg protein, soy protein, sugars and flavouring. Vegetable gums are often added to give body to the drink (not you). They are usually expensive and the ingredient list is impressively long. However, if you check out the amino acid content of protein supplements you will find that they are very similar to many protein rich foods.

If you purchased a certain expensive brand of popular protein powder the recommended serving size is 30 grams, several times per day. Only 9 grams of those 30 grams contain protein. However, if you decided to make your own protein powder with skim milk powder, the same 9grams protein would only set you back 13 cents.

The Table below shows a comparison of what you would get if you had $1.00 to spend on protein.

Food	Protein	Food	Protein
165g Skim Milk Powder	60g	150g Tuna in Brine	35g
83g Skinless Baked Chicken	25g	35g Popular Brand Protein Powder	9g

It is worthwhile remembering that your body cannot tell the difference between expensive protein powders and those made in your kitchen.

57. Are carbohydrates fattening?

Simply put: consuming an excess of food energy (calories or kilojoules) in any form (carbohydrate, fat, protein or alcohol) and not getting enough exercise will increase your body fat.

Carbohydrate is found in bread, cereal, pasta, rice, some fruit, potatoes, sweet potatoes, corn, milk, yoghurt, legumes, sugar, honey and lollies. All carbohydrates get broken down into glucose and are absorbed into the bloodstream.

Once carbohydrate is digested and broken down into glucose, it is very efficiently stored as glycogen in the muscles and liver. It is possible, albeit difficult, to eat excess carbohydrate (more than 800 grams per day) and so your body reacts by using this excess as fuel and then stores any fat that you eat as body fat.

For example, 800 grams of carbohydrate is equivalent to 12 Weet-bix™, 5 bananas, 10 slices of bread, 4 cups of pasta, 10 scoops of ice cream and 1 litre of fruit juice. Not just one of these foods but the combination of them all equates to 800 grams of carbohydrate. Unless you are a hard-training athlete, consuming this amount is no easy feat!

You need to be aware of the fat that may be associated with foods containing carbohydrate e.g. cakes and biscuits. Some carbohydrates are very easy to consume in large quantities because they are low in fibre and contain little bulk to make you feel full. Some examples of these are soft drinks, fruit juice, sugar in coffee and tea, and lollies.

Try sitting down with 86 potatoes and eating them all in one go - this is the amount you would have to eat to gain 1kg in body weight! Carbohydrates are not the villains in the weight war; it is what is added to them, like fats and sugars, which are the real bad guys.

58. Are muscle cramps caused by a lack of salt?

This is somewhat unknown. Many people have experienced the gripping pain of a sudden cramp, which most often occurs in the calf muscle or the foot. Cramps most commonly occur during exercise but can also affect stationary muscles. It is known that cramp is due to an involuntary muscle contraction, but the reasons for cramps are not clear-cut. Cramps may be partly due to dehydration, muscle overload, fatigue, heavy salt losses or extremes of temperature. It is commonly thought that a cure for muscle cramps is taking salt or salt tablets. There is a small minority of athletes or individuals who may lose large amounts of sodium (salt) in their sweat, possibly leading to cramps. However, it is not wise to take salt tablets as they make dehydration worse by drawing water from the blood stream into the intestine, increasing the risk of further dehydration.

Sports Dietitians Australia (SDA) is a professional organisation of Dietitians specialising in the field of sports nutrition and they recommend several steps that you can take to reduce the risk of cramp. They include:

- Be fit. Cramps are less common in athletes who are well trained.
- Drink plenty of fluids before, during and after exercise or physical work to avoid dehydration.

- Eat well and cut down on the fats that clog arteries. Cramps occur in muscles that have a reduced blood supply due to narrowed arteries.
- Stretch before and after exercise. If you suffer night cramps, stretch before going to bed.
- Wear proper clothing. Loose comfortable clothes are best. Tight fitting clothes can reduce blood flow to muscles making them more susceptible to cramps.
- Acclimatise to warmer weather to help avoid dehydration.

59. Are sports drinks high in sugar and salt?

Sports drinks actually contain less sugar than soft drinks but should only be used before, during and after extended bouts of exercise. Carbohydrate-containing fluids such as sports drinks address both the fluid and carbohydrate needs of an athlete. Most good sports drinks contain between 4-8% carbohydrate and act to delay fatigue by sparing muscle glycogen stores and topping up blood glucose. Adding glucose and sodium (salt) increases the absorption of water and sports drinks are most beneficial for exercise lasting for 1 hour or longer. In relation to dental decay, scientific research shows that sports drinks are no greater culprit than any other carbohydrate-containing food or drink.

There has been some concern from the general public that sports drinks are too salty and may increase the risk of high blood pressure. It's important to realise that sports drinks were not originally targeted at the sedentary population at large. There are people who go to the local deli and choose a sports drink because it makes them feel 'sporty'. Believe it or not this is not the same as being active, even if the advertising is trying to convince you otherwise! The Australian Dietary Guidelines do recommend a reduction in salt intake, but the salt level of sports drinks is approximately equal to that found in milk and this level generally does not pose a significant health problem.

60. Does eating an orange prevent muscle cramp during sport?

In Australian sporting culture the orange (cut into quarters) has long been a part of weekend sport and something to look forward to at half- time. Given that the reasons for cramps are not clear-cut, it is not feasible to suggest that eating an orange will prevent them from happening. However, eating an orange will provide you with some fluid, Vitamin C, and a small amount of carbohydrate (an average orange contains approximately 110 mL of water and 10 grams carbohydrate) so go ahead and enjoy one!

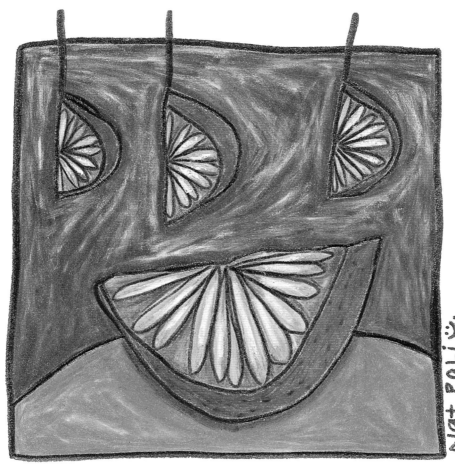

61. Can athletes drink more alcohol than the average person because they will 'sweat it off' the next day?

In short - no. On average your body can metabolise one standard drink of alcohol per hour through your liver. This does depend on quite a few factors including age, gender, body mass, drinking experience and food eaten and may be more or less accurate, accordingly. This is true of athletes and non-athletes alike.

It is true that after a heavy drinking session you can often smell alcohol on one's body, but it is generally bad breath, not alcohol being excreted through sweat. In the mid 1980s, two sports medicine experts made an interesting assessment on the nutritional knowledge of a group of elite athletes in Australia. Twenty-six percent of the athletes believed that alcohol contained no kilojoules, reduced inhibition and actually improved their performance. Wrong!

It would be interesting to see how much that perception has changed but given that the sports culture in Australia still encourages alcohol consumption in the name of team spirit and friendship, perhaps the change has not been significant.

62. Are energy drinks the same as sports drinks?

No. 'Energy drinks' should not be confused with common 'Sports drinks' such as Gatorade®, Powerade® and others which were originally developed for athletes.

Energy drinks such as Red Bull®, V™ and Mother® have flooded the market in the last few years and primarily appeal to weekend athletes, children and teenagers. They contain a wide range of ingredients including sugar, caffeine and/or guarana, B-group vitamins, amino acids and herbal products. Sugar is the main carbohydrate and energy source, and its concentration is often 11-15% in these products. This level of carbohydrate is similar to cordials and soft drinks but significantly higher than sports drinks. The high sugar concentration can slow your stomach emptying and affect fluid absorption. There is little scientific evidence to prove the addition of amino acids (such as taurine), or herbal ingredients (like ginseng) to energy drinks are beneficial.

The main ingredient of interest in energy drinks for most people is caffeine. Caffeine is a stimulant that affects the brain, nervous system, heart, kidneys, muscles and lungs. Despite marketing claims to the contrary, guarana contains caffeine and acts in exactly the same way.

Most authorities agree that the safe daily upper limit for caffeine is 300mg for the average adult person and there is no safe limit for children. 300mg is equivalent to 3-4 cups of brewed coffee (cappuccino, latte, flat white etc).

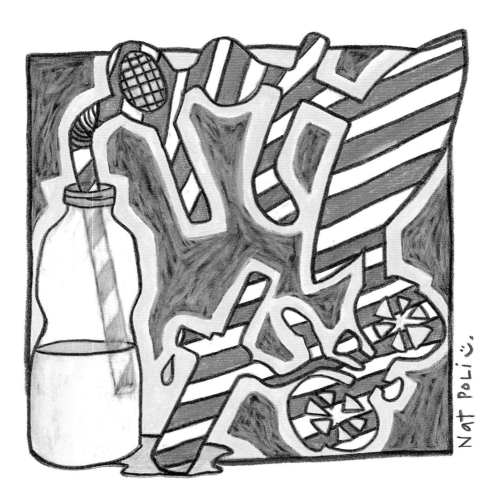

Nat Poli.

Energy drinks are not a good choice for fluid replacement during sport and should not replace sports drinks or water. Scientific evidence has shown repeatedly that sports drinks provide a performance benefit in exercise lasting longer than 1 hour. Sports drinks contain between 6-8% carbohydrate and some electrolytes including sodium (salt). These ingredients promote the absorption of fluid and carbohydrates during exercise.

When choosing a drink before, during and after exercise, sports drinks or water are the best choices.

63. Does muscle convert into fat when you stop exercising?

Thankfully, no. When you jump on the scales, the number that you see is a combination of a number of things including blood, bone, water, muscle and fat. Essentially think of the human body as a mass made up of fat and muscle. They are separate components and cannot transform from one to the other. If you stop exercising, you will lose muscle tone and bulk, but the muscle itself does not get converted into fat.

It is worth noting that muscle does weigh more than fat, so after exercising for some time an increase on the scales might occur. However, this can only be a good thing as muscle controls your metabolic rate. The greater percentage of muscle in the body, the higher your metabolic rate and the more efficient your body is at burning fuel and therefore fat.

64. If I exercise regularly should I take a nutrition supplement?

Some supplements may be useful when trying to improve your workout performance but you should always first look at what you are eating. The greatest nutritional benefits are often found in your everyday diet! Eating a varied and balanced diet regularly will provide most of the nutrition your body requires.

There is a vast array of nutritional supplements on the market and the industry is worth billions of dollars each year. There are a few categories of dietary supplements, which include:

- Those similar to normal food – liquid meals such as Sustagen® Sport and Up and Go® drinks
- Special formulations – sports drinks, high carbohydrate supplements, multi-vitamins and minerals and specific vitamins and minerals
- Nutritional ergogenic aids – contains nutrients or other food components in amounts far greater than the recommended dietary intake or amounts present in food

If you are considering using supplements, do your research thoroughly and seek the advice of a Sports Dietitian.

65. Does caffeine help the body break down fat for energy?

This seems to be a common belief. However, the evidence is mixed in regards to whether caffeine breaks down fat for energy, so the answer to the question is maybe!

There is much interest in caffeine amongst athletes, coaches and health professionals as a possible performance-enhancing drug. There is also interest in whether it has a role in utilising fat stores for fuel. A series of investigations 30 years ago found that a moderate intake of caffeine one hour before exercise increased the use of fat stores for energy. Researchers also found that the consumption of caffeine resulted in carbohydrate stores (glycogen) being spared, meaning that the body should be able to exercise longer. Other, more recent studies have found that caffeine consumption increases adrenaline levels. Adrenaline improves alertness and reaction times and it is thought by some experts to enhance the use of fat as a fuel.

However, not all researchers agree with this theory, and there may be several ways that caffeine could affect these responses.

It is worthwhile remembering that individual responses to caffeine differ greatly and until more research is conducted no firm recommendations can be made.

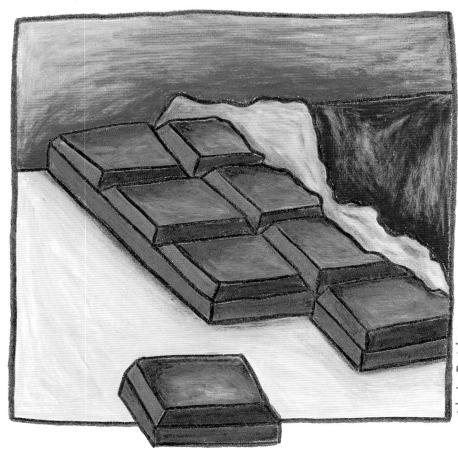

66. Should I eat a Mars Bar® prior to playing a game of football (or other sport)?

No. Mars Bars® have a medium Glycemic Index (GI) of 62 and contain 10 grams of fat. Fat slows down the emptying of the stomach and therefore digestion and these factors combined mean that Mars Bars® are best enjoyed at a time not associated with exercise.

Some of you will remember the television advertisement that was aired in the 1980s for Mars Bars®. The ad jingle contained lyrics suggesting that Mars Bars® helped you 'work, rest and play'. There was definitely a sports theme to the advertisement and over time, this has led to the belief that Mars Bars® are a good pre-game snack. Great advertising – but not so great for your body!

Any pre-workout snack or meal should provide you with sustained energy to perform the activity to the best of your ability, and be easily digested. The food should be predominantly carbohydrate with a small amount of protein and minimal fat. Ideally the food should be of low to medium Glycemic Index (refer to Question 14 for a summary) and consumed 1 ½ to 2 hours prior to the event.

Some healthy low fat pre-game snacks include: cereal and milk, toast with baked beans or spaghetti, bread or toast with low fat spread, Up and Go® drink or Sustagen® Sport, creamed rice and fruit and low fat muesli bars.

67. Is it possible to maintain energy levels for exercise whilst trying to reduce body weight?

Yes it is. During most exercise your body will burn a fuel mix of carbohydrate and fat, and the amount will depend on the intensity and length of the exercise session. When trying to reduce body weight we are essentially trying to burn off our fat stores.

Some people make the mistake of reducing their food intake to the extent that they have no energy to exercise and are eating very little carbohydrate. Carbohydrates provide your body with the fuel to exercise, and reducing or eliminating these from your diet can be very counterproductive to weight loss. Remember that often, fat is the culprit as it is stored more efficiently in the body than either protein or carbohydrate. Reducing dietary fat intake is one of the most effective strategies in promoting weight loss! Some guidelines that may help include:

- Choose a percentage body fat or weight that is healthy and achievable without stress on your body.
- Review what you are eating and remember that the basis for weight loss is very simple. What goes in (food) must be less than what goes out (exercise). Don't starve yourself.
- Choose a balanced diet that is low in fat. Carbohydrate is essential for exercise but don't overdo that either. Remember that it is the total calories that count.
- Seek professional advice from an Accredited Practising Dietitian on specific dietary requirements and realistic weight goals.

- If you are exercising for longer than 1 hour you will need to consume some carbohydrate and a small amount of protein. For snack and meal ideas in relation to sport, check out www.sportsdietitians.com.

68. Is it usual for my body weight to be higher at the end of the day in comparison to the beginning?

Yes. Some people find that their body weight differs, sometimes significantly, from morning to night. It is likely that you will be lightest first thing in the morning before breakfast because you have had nothing to eat or drink for several hours. As the day wears on, body fluid may increase due to food and fluid intake and be reflected in an increase on the scales. But this is not permanent and is gone again the next morning. Of course, if you are eating more than you need to on a regular basis, extra weight may become a permanent fixture.

69. Should pregnant women avoid fish?

Some fish contain mercury levels that may harm an unborn baby or young child's developing nervous system. Mercury is a naturally occurring element that is found in air, water and food - most people are exposed to it through food. Fish ingest mercury from streams and oceans as they feed and it binds to their tissue proteins (such as muscle). Food processing, preparation and cooking techniques don't significantly reduce the amount of mercury in fish.

The good news is that you can receive all the benefits of eating fish while pregnant or planning to become pregnant (within a 6 month period) if some simple dietary advice is followed. One serving is considered to be 150 grams. Some tips to consider are:

- Avoid fish with high levels of mercury such as shark, swordfish, barramundi, gem fish, orange roughy (deep sea perch), ling and southern blue fin tuna.
- Limit other fish, such as tuna steaks, to one serve per week or three 95g cans of tuna per week (smaller tuna contain less mercury).

There are no limits on the intake of fresh or tinned salmon and fortunately, most fish in Australia have low mercury levels.

70. Do particular foods cause cancer?

Much research has been conducted to work out whether there is a link between what we eat and cancer. Some of the research is not final but a number of links have been found. Some of the findings are:

- There is much controversy regarding red meat and colorectal cancer. The current evidence is weak and inconclusive on fresh red meat, but a stronger association has been found with processed meats such as salami, ham and bacon.
- Fruit and vegetables may lower the risk of developing cancers of the digestive tract.
- Diets very high in salt have been linked to an increased risk of developing stomach cancer. This is particularly relevant to people who eat diets high in foods that are pickled, salted or smoked. Japan and Korea are notable examples of this problem.
- There is overwhelming evidence to suggest that being overweight or obese increases the risk of developing cancer, especially that of the bowel, breast, oesophagus, endometrium (womb) and pancreas. Eating a healthy diet and exercising regularly will reduce the risk of becoming overweight and obese.

So, in practical terms what does this mean in our daily lives? Some tips from the cancer council are:

- Eat at least 2 servings of fruit and 5 servings of vegetables every day
- Choose wholegrain breads and cereals

- Limit intake of processed meats and avoid high temperature cooking and charring of red meat
- Limit saturated and trans fats
- Minimise salty food and avoid adding salt to food
- Maintain a healthy body weight and keep physically active

For more information on nutrition and cancer click on www.cancerwa.asn.au.

71. Does red meat cause cancer?

Lately, the role of meat in the diet has been controversial. In 2002 the International Agency for Research on Cancer published an analysis on the relationship between meat consumption and colorectal cancer. At this time, fresh meat appears to be unrelated to the risk of colorectal cancer. An increased risk of colorectal cancer was associated with an increased consumption of processed meats like ham, bacon, salami, sausages and frankfurts (hot dogs). The Cancer Council recommends that we limit our intake of such processed meats, which are high in fat, salt and nitrates.

Until more conclusive evidence is available it is advisable to avoid char-grilling, reduce high temperature cooking of meat (pan-frying) and use more roasting, stewing and microwaving.

72. Do artificial sweeteners give you cancer?

No. There are different types of artificial sweeteners including saccharin, cyclamate and most commonly, aspartame. Aspartame is actually a combination of two amino acids, which are linked together to produce a sweet taste. One of the amino acids that aspartame breaks down into is phenylalanine. Phenylalanine is one of the 'essential' amino acids and has to be obtained through food, as the body can't manufacture it.

One of the most common questions that I get asked is, "are diet soft drinks safe to drink and what harm will phenylalanine do?"

Amino acids are the building blocks of protein and these amino acids are found naturally in many protein containing foods including meat, dairy products, legumes and grains. When our bodies break down aspartame, it digests the amino acid components in exactly the same way it digests these components from food.

"Please be aware that this product contains phenylalanine" is a warning that is legally required on every product sweetened with aspartame. The manufacturers are warning those people with a disease known as phenylketonuria, because they cannot digest this amino acid normally and consuming it will result in severe medical problems. This warning is not applicable to many of us as we can digest and absorb phenylalanine without any problem.

Aspartame has been commercially available since 1983, is found in over 100 countries and used in more than 6000 products worldwide. All sweeteners available in Australia have passed stringent tests by FSANZ (Food Standards Australia and New Zealand) to ensure that they are safe. There is a lot of misinformation regarding artificial sweeteners available on the Internet, most of which is debatable.

The good thing about artificial sweeteners is that they are not sugar and contain virtually no kilojoules. They are 180-200 times sweeter than sugar, so only a small amount is needed. Another point to consider is the ADI or Acceptable Daily Intake. This is the amount of a food additive that can be ingested over an entire lifetime without any appreciable risk to health.

For a 70kg adult to reach the ADI when using aspartame they would need to consume 184 tablets or 220 teaspoons of aspartame spoon for spoon every day over their lifetime. No easy feat!

73. Does food acidity or alkalinity have any impact on our health?

The acidity and alkalinity of food are physical properties that may alter the rate of emptying of the stomach, digestion in the small bowel and the acidity/alkalinity of our urine. However, these two properties do not present any issue for our bodies. Acidic foods generally have an acid flavour while alkaline foods might taste slightly soapy.

74. Is microwaving food dangerous?

No. Extensive research has provided no substantiated evidence that microwave exposure, at any level, either causes or promotes cancer. Microwaves generated in microwave ovens cease to exist once the electrical power is turned off. They do not remain in the food when taken out of the microwave oven. Neither can they make the food or the oven radioactive. Therefore, food cooked in a microwave oven is not a radiation hazard.

It would be difficult today to find a household that does not have a microwave oven. This is for good reason as they are convenient, quick and can be used for all types of food. The microwaves penetrate the food and agitate the water molecules within. This causes molecular friction, which produces heat and results in a rapid rise in temperature. The microwaves produced while cooking heat the water in food so that the cooking process is similar to steam cooking.

Water-soluble vitamins including Vitamin C are the main nutrients likely to be lost during the cooking of fruit and vegetables. Vitamin C is also heat soluble and this means that if the cooking time is reduced and minimal water used, then greater amounts of that vitamin will be retained. Microwave cooking addresses both of these issues as the cooking time required is short and minimal amounts of water are needed. Generally speaking, microwave cooking retains nutrients as well as, if not better than, conventional methods.

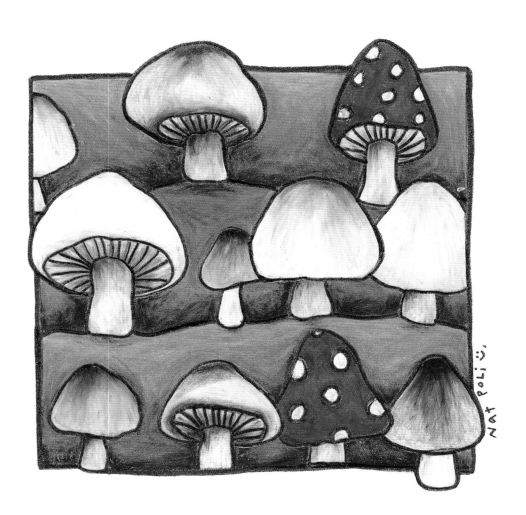

Nat Poli

75. Are mushrooms a good source of Vitamin B12?

Mushrooms do contain a small amount of Vitamin B12 but one serving of this will provide you with only 5% of the Recommended Daily Intake (RDI). However they do contain other nutrients such as Vitamin B, selenium, copper and fibre.

Vitamin B12 plays a role in the formation of genetic material in DNA, which is an important chemical involved in protein production. A deficiency in Vitamin B12 results in anaemia and abnormal working of the central nervous system. When the body can't absorb Vitamin B12 properly it can cause a condition called pernicious anaemia, which is not the fault of one's diet. Injections of the vitamin are given in that situation.

Vitamin B12 is primarily found in animal products and if you are eating these foods you are unlikely to suffer any deficiency. Due to their supposed Vitamin B12 content, mushrooms are often incorrectly promoted as the vegetarians' alternative to meat.

76. Is organic food better for you than conventionally produced food?

Unproven. The nutritional superiority of organic food is often touted; however, there is no scientific evidence to support such claims. Consumers do perceive organic food to be healthier than conventional food, despite insufficient evidence to support this view. Some reports have shown the protein content to be lower and the content of Vitamin C and some minerals and phytochemicals to be higher in organic food. However, these studies have been unreliable. Reviews of the broader scientific literature indicate that there is little or no difference in the nutrient content of foods that are produced by organic or conventional methods.

The organic food industry is growing at a fast pace worldwide and it is predicted that by 2016, 30% of Australia's food will be organic.

The issue of pesticides is a factor that encourages people to purchase organic foods over conventional. Organic produce could contain pesticide residue as a result of contamination from neighbouring conventional farms and some organic farms may use botanical pesticides. The levels of pesticide residues are generally lower in organic produce however, the levels of pesticide in conventional produce are already much lower than the acceptable daily intake set by the Australian Pesticide and Veterinary Medicines Authority.

77. Are probiotics good for your health?

The scientifically established benefits of probiotics are:

- Prevention or reduction of the duration of rotavirus diarrhoea
- Prevention or reduction of the duration of antibiotic associated diarrhoea
- Reduction of the symptoms of lactose intolerance

Other benefits have been suggested, however there is a need for further research with probiotic bacteria in relation to:

- Bladder and colon cancer (prevention and treatment)
- Inflammatory Bowel Disease
- Food Allergy
- Irritable Bowel Syndrome
- Cholesterol control

Probiotics are foods or supplements that contain live beneficial bacteria that help to improve the overall balance of bacteria in the digestive system. There are a number of sources including fermented milk drinks (e.g. Yakult®), yoghurts, capsules and powders.

Stress, diet, aging and antibiotics may upset our intestinal balance and probiotics may be especially useful during these times. And no, we can't stop the aging process but we can impact the other factors.

Be aware that some fermented milks arrive in store frozen and this appears to render the bacteria ineffective. This can be the case for some store brand varieties of fermented milk. Choice magazine tested the viability of bacteria in probiotics' over time in 1999 and found that Yakult®, Vaalia® Smoothie, Vaalia® Yoghurt and Yoplus® Light all showed good survivability of bacteria over the shelf life. This is the most recent survey to date. Yakult® contains one of the highest levels of bacteria at 100 million bacteria per ml.

Supplements in liquid, capsule or powder form may carry high levels of bacteria but they are not live. They should also be refrigerated which is not often the case in pharmacies and health food stores.

78. Is it true that we need to eat a lot of fibre to keep healthy?

Basically, fibre is essential to good health and works to:

- Relieve constipation
- Help fight cancer: Fibre dilutes the bowel contents and shortens the time for food residue to pass through the large intestine, which minimises contact with any carcinogens (cancer-causing substances). It also has the ability to bind possible cancer agents and excrete them. 1 in 12 Australians will be diagnosed with bowel cancer by the age of 85, so increasing fibre intake and decreasing fat intake has the potential to significantly improve bowel health in Australia.

- Lower cholesterol: Soluble fibres such as oat bran, barley bran, rice bran, pectin, guar gum, psyllium and many dried beans have been shown to lower cholesterol, particularly LDL.
- Improve diabetic control: Fibre slows down the absorption of nutrients and lowers the Glycemic Index, so nutrients, especially glucose, are absorbed into the bloodstream slowly.

Many people think that a high fibre diet is "rabbit food" and is often characterised as consisting of twigs, leaves and birdseed! Rest assured it is not.

When you are not used to eating a high fibre diet and you increase your fibre intake, you may not be very popular with friends until your body adjusts! But this extra 'wind' your body is producing is normal and healthy.

We need 30 grams of fibre every day. Try the following:

- Fruits and vegetables - where possible leave the skin on. Try to eat at least 2 servings of fruit (1 serve = 1 whole piece or 1 cup) per day and 5 servings of vegetables (1 serve = ½ cup).
- Bread - wholegrain and wholemeal are higher in fibre than white bread and should be your first choice. You might like to try white hyfibe bread if you don't like wholemeal.
- Breakfast cereals - these can be hard to pick but go for the less processed varieties and choose those with greater than 10 grams of fibre per 100 grams cereal. Bran-based cereals are high in fibre but highly processed cereals such as Cornflakes and Rice-bubbles® contain little fibre.

- Legumes - this group includes lentils, chickpeas and kidney beans and any dried bean (including canned such as baked beans) and they are very high in fibre.
- Grains - rice, pasta, cracked wheat, oats, barley, rye and millet are good sources of fibre. Wholemeal varieties of rice and pasta contain more fibre than white varieties.
- Nuts and seeds - good source of fibre and are acceptable in small amounts but they also contain considerable amounts of fat.

To meet your daily fibre need of 30 grams, here is an example of what to eat:

- 1 cup of high fibre breakfast cereal
- 3 slices of wholegrain bread
- 3 servings of fruit
- 5 servings of vegetables

Of course, you can select your own individual preferences.

79. Can drinking water cure migraines or headaches?

It can't hurt! There is no research to suggest that drinking water will cure a migraine but one symptom of dehydration or lack of fluid is a headache. Migraines are a complex medical problem and the trigger factors are varied depending on the individual. Cheese, chocolate and oranges may sound like a gourmet delight but these foods have been linked to the pain of migraine. Although some sufferers cite food as a trigger for their migraine or headache, much of the evidence linking diet and migraine is unsound and as yet unproven.

So, rather than curing the problem it may be easier to prevent the onset of a headache by ensuring that your fluid intake is regular, particularly when exercising.

80. Does certain food cause acne?

Possibly! The link between diet and acne has been tenuous at best for some time until recently when a study was conducted by researchers at the RMIT University in Melbourne. They investigated the effect of diet on two groups of men aged 15-25 years over 3 months.

One group ate a typical Western diet containing highly processed foods such as white bread, biscuits and chips. The other group ate a higher protein, low glycemic index diet containing fresh fruits, vegetables, lean red meat, chicken, seafood and whole grains. Processed and takeaway foods were kept to a minimum and this eating plan became known as the Anti-Acne Diet.

The Anti-Acne Diet was found to reduce acne by more than 50% over the 12 weeks. Some of the healthier choices made during this study were:

Western Diet	Anti-Acne Diet
High sugar ready-to-eat cereals	High fibre cereals, rolled oats and natural muesli
White or wholemeal bread	Grainy bread, sourdough or fruit loaf
White rice	Basmati or Doongara rice, pasta, fresh noodles
Crackers	Grainy crispbreads
Sugar	Honey
Biscuits, cake, lollies, muesli bars	Fresh fruit, vegetables, dried fruit, unsalted nuts, seeds, low fat dairy foods
Crisps	Plain popcorn
Potatoes	Sweet potato, sweet corn or carrots
Soft drink	Water, low fat milk, fruit juice

Protein rich foods such as red meat, poultry, fish and eggs were also part of the package and the research has indicated that they are integral for healthy skin and should be consumed at each meal. Regular exercise is important also.

While this study has made some significant findings, further research is required.

For more information on the Glycemic Index see Question 14 and checkout www.glycemicindex.com. For further information on the Anti-Acne Diet see www.themainmeal.com.au or call 1800 550 018 for a copy.

81. Is the information on a food label helpful when choosing a healthy diet?

Absolutely. Food labels can be very helpful when making supermarket choices. The information is there, so use it to your advantage to choose healthier food. In December 2000, Australian and New Zealand Health Ministers decided to improve food labels and that process was completed in December 2002. Food labelling laws are governed by the food standards code, which is administered by the Food Standards Australia and New Zealand (FSANZ).

The type of information that you will find on a food label includes the following:

- Name or description of the food
- Nutrition information panel
- Ingredients list
- Manufacturer details
- Storage requirements
- Date marking
- Product weight
- Possible nutrition claim
- Information for allergy sufferers

The ingredient list can be very useful because the items are listed from the largest to the smallest volume. A product high in fat or sugar would have these listed in the first few ingredients.

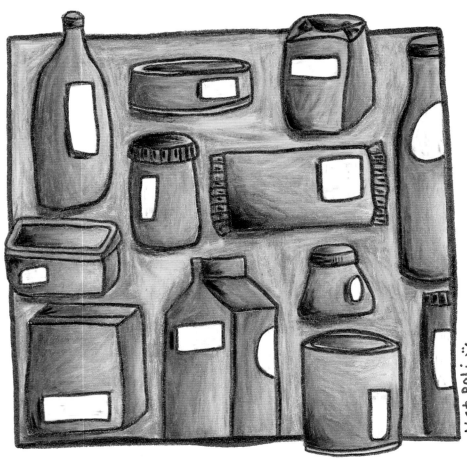

Nat Poli ☺.

The most specific information can be found on the nutrition information panel. The food standards code requires the manufacturer to include:

- Energy
- Protein
- Total fat
- Saturated fat
- Total carbohydrate
- Sugars
- Sodium (salt)
- Country of origin

The nutrition information panel may also include calcium, fibre and other vitamins and minerals, if the product is a good source of the nutrient or the manufacturer has made a claim about the particular nutrient.

The label may also include a nutrition claim such as:

- No added sugar
- Low fat
- Reduced fat
- Low salt
- 97% fat free or cholesterol free
- Lite or light

These claims have to be backed up by information in the nutrition panel. For example; for a product to be considered 'low fat' it must not contain more than 3 grams of total fat per 100 grams of the product. It is considered to be reduced fat if the product contains 8 grams or less of total fat per 100 grams of the product.

For a Virtual Supermarket Tour, checkout www.daa.asn.au and click on 'Smart Eating for You'. Once in this section you will be able to do the 'Tour' and hone your label reading skills. The Diabetes Association in your state conducts Shop Smart Supermarket tours, check the internet for details.

The following quote sums up the food labelling experience.

"Knowing and not doing is the same as not knowing." - Anon

82. What does the National Heart Foundation Tick mean?

The 'Tick' is the Heart Foundation's guide to help people make healthy food choices quickly and easily. Every food carrying the Heart Foundation Tick has passed independent tests to ensure strict nutrition standards have been met – no exceptions. There are more than 60 different food categories with Tick alternatives, each with their own criteria for combinations of saturated fat, salt, kilojoules and fibre.

Over one third of the products in the Tick program are fresh foods. All fresh fruit and vegetables automatically get the Tick. The Tick can also appear on foods that are high in fat, like margarines, oils and nuts. These products have had the saturated fat content lowered and the content of unsaturated or healthier fats increased proportionately.

An example of a high fat food earning the Tick would be McDonalds® Australia fast food restaurants. In 2007 McDonalds® launched nine Tick-approved meals that are served in their restaurants across the country. These meals meet the Tick's strict standards for serving size, saturated fat, salt and vegetable/fibre content. It is interesting to note that the recipe changes at McDonalds® have resulted in the removal of 2585 kilograms of salt annually from the Australian food supply.

Tick products are subject to random testing and failure to meet the guidelines can result in that company's product being expelled from the Tick Program. Food companies do pay a royalty fee and this is based on the wholesale turnover of their Tick product. This means that smaller companies with smaller turnovers are not disadvantaged. Approximately half of the companies in the Tick program pay the minimum annual royalty fee of $2000.00. The National Heart Foundation is a non-profit, non-government organisation and the royalty fee is used to run the Tick program.

While the 'Tick' can help you make good food choices, it does not mean that you can eat unlimited quantities of a particular food. Nor does it mean that food without the 'Tick' symbol is necessarily 'bad' for you.

83. Can eating too much salt cause high blood pressure?

A research group called the Dietary Approaches to Stop Hypertension (DASH) instigated a clinical trial that required participants to consume a controlled diet for 8 weeks. Participants ate either a typical Western diet, a fruit and vegetable diet or a combination diet known as the DASH diet. This trial showed that a diet rich in fruit and vegetables and low fat dairy products could reduce blood pressure in the general population and people with Stage 1 Hypertension.

This original DASH diet did not require either salt restriction or weight loss. There has since been a follow-up study to DASH, called DASH-sodium that has demonstrated a reduction in salt intake in combination with the DASH diet is even more effective.

High blood pressure or hypertension occurs when blood vessels harden leading to a build-up of pressure. It increases the risk of developing heart disease and stroke and can lead to problems in other parts of the body such as the eyes and kidneys.

So, to reduce blood pressure consider the following:

- Eat less salt (sodium)
- Drink less alcohol
- Avoid smoking
- Maintain a healthy body weight
- Eat a diet rich in fruit and vegetables

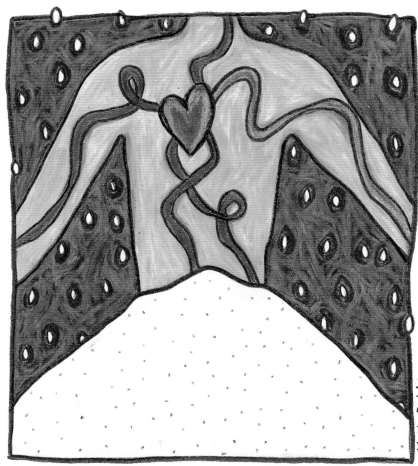

Nat Polic.

84. Are all types of salt the same?

Salt is a chemical compound of sodium and chlorine and is called sodium chloride. Rock and sea salt are almost entirely sodium chloride with only traces of other minerals. Iodised salt contains approximately 0.03 milligrams of iodine per gram of salt and is intended as a supplement for people whose diet is deficient in iodine. This is relevant to the Australian population as evidence of mild iodine deficiency emerged in Australia and New Zealand in the late 1990s. Adequate iodine is essential for the brain development of unborn babies, infants and young children. Iodine is only found in small quantities in food and iodised salt is the richest source available. Iodine aside, all types of salt contains the same quantity of sodium chloride and are therefore nutritionally equal.

85. Is vegetable protein the same as animal protein?

No. While animal and plant foods both provide protein, they are not the same. Protein is an essential nutrient for our bodies and is made up of amino acids. Like Lego®, lots of blocks form a house, and lots of amino acids strung together form proteins. Some of these amino acids are essential and are found only in food; and others are non-essential and manufactured by the body. Foods with proteins that do not contain all of the essential amino acids are known as incomplete protein foods while foods that contain proteins with all the essential amino acids are called complete proteins.

Generally speaking, protein from animal foods is complete while protein from vegetable sources is incomplete. For vegetarians, this can present a problem. Incomplete proteins can be complementary to each other and combined to form complete proteins. Some years ago it was thought that vegetarians needed to combine particular types of incomplete proteins in the same meal for this effect to occur. Scientists now know that as long as a number of incomplete proteins are consumed during the course of a day, this will result in the same effect.

Some examples of protein foods are below:

Incomplete Protein Foods
- Grains – rice, corn, bread, oats, pasta and breakfast cereals
- Legumes – good old baked beans, kidney beans, chickpeas, cannellini and borlotti beans
- Nuts and seeds

Complete Protein Foods
- Meat, chicken and fish
- Dairy products – milk, cheese and yoghurt
- Eggs

Animal protein foods are richer in some nutrients such as iron, calcium and zinc; and a greater percentage is available for absorption by the body in comparison to vegetable protein. In addition, lower calorie diets need a greater percentage of protein to ensure nutrient needs are met.

This means that vegetarians should be diligent with their food choices to ensure optimal nutritional status.

86. Is eating breakfast important to our well-being?

Yes! The most important thing about breakfast is that you actually eat it. It is the first meal of the day and the term 'breakfast' is an English word meaning to 'break the fast'. Many people do not eat breakfast and the most common reason is a lack of time. Make time!

Most nutritionists consider it the most important meal of the day and are supported by many research studies. In 2005, researchers reviewed the results of 47 studies that looked at the association of breakfast consumption with nutritional adequacy, body weight and academic performance in children and adolescents. The evidence suggests that eating breakfast can improve memory, school results and school attendance - as well as having a positive impact on general health and well-being.

In addition, those children who ate breakfast consistently consumed more daily calories but were less likely to be overweight. Adults can gain the same benefits from eating breakfast.
So what should you choose? Pick a breakfast that is high in fibre and low in fat and above all, tasty. Some ideas for a healthy breakfast include:

- High fibre cereal with low fat milk or yoghurt and fruit
- Low fat yoghurt with fresh or tinned fruit
- Pancakes with fresh fruit
- Tinned spaghetti or baked beans on wholegrain toast
- Low fat fruit smoothie
- Wholegrain toast with jam, honey, peanut butter or Vegemite®
- Poached, scrambled or boiled eggs on a toasted English muffin
- Mushrooms, grilled tomato or sweet corn on wholegrain toast

87. Should you take multi-vitamins to support your diet?

Complementary medicine like vitamin and mineral supplementation does have a place in our health and well-being, but it is best to focus on fine-tuning your diet before turning to supplements. There is no need to use them as a back up unless you are part of a nutritionally compromised group such as the elderly, pregnant or breastfeeding women.

The multi-vitamin industry is worth billions of dollars worldwide annually. In 2006 in Australia alone, the dietary supplement industry was worth $1.1 billion.

It is very difficult to overdose on vitamins and minerals through the food we eat daily, since these nutrients are only one component of the food. Supplements are a different story and one must be careful with them. Vitamins are classified as either fat or water-soluble. The fat-soluble vitamins are A, D, E and K and they are stored in our fat depots. This means that their stores can accumulate and an overdose of these vitamins can be toxic. Any excess water-soluble vitamins are excreted in the urine, which prevents toxicity.

Although the safety of vitamins and minerals is monitored closely in Australia, the effectiveness of these supplements is not regulated. They are generally not allowed to make health claims on their labelling but it can still be very difficult for the consumer to make a decision.

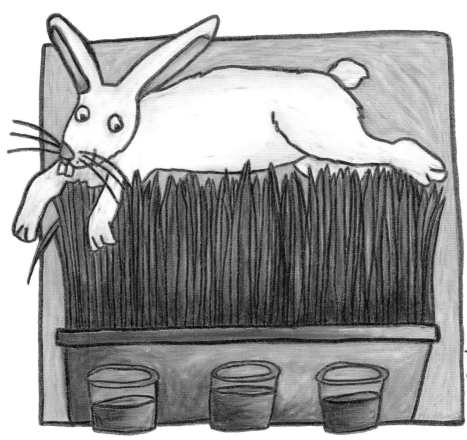

Nat Polić.

88. Is a wheatgrass shot good for my health?

Wheatgrass is the bright green display that you often see at juicing bars. It is a type of grass and costs around $2.40 per 30ml shot. The taste is interesting to say the least and not an experience I personally feel the need to repeat. (Thankfully the wheatgrass was served with an orange wedge, which did help to eradicate the taste.)

Wheatgrass has many supposed health benefits associated with its use and its supporters claim that it:

- Improves the digestive system
- Prevents cancer, diabetes and heart disease
- Cures constipation
- Detoxifies heavy metals from the bloodstream
- Cleanses the liver
- Prevents hair loss
- Helps make menopause more manageable
- Promotes general well-being

In summary, it sounds like a miracle food! It is worth noting that none of these claims have been substantiated in scientific literature and the proposed benefits are unproven. Based on this, wheatgrass is not recommended unless you particularly like the taste and don't mind paying for it.

89. Is there a connection between hormones in chicken and 'man-boobs' (or human breast development)?

This potential link does not exist, as thankfully, hormones have been banned from poultry feed in Australia for over 35 years. This is backed up by results from the National Residue Survey, which monitors hormone residues in Australian poultry meat products and ensures they are absent.

Australians eat quite a bit of chicken. There are 428 million chickens slaughtered in Australia annually for meat production. A common misconception surrounding chicken meat is that the manufacturers feed poultry hormones to stimulate quicker growth and that it could be linked to human breast development. Public opinion deems that this is not considered to be a problem for women, but in men, 'man-boobs' are not so popular. Generally, too much body fat and un-toned pectoral muscles are to blame for this condition.

90. Does drinking water during a meal hinder digestion?

No. The premise behind this theory is that water dilutes the gastric juices required to digest our food. Fortunately this is not the case, and in fact water can actually aid rather than hinder the digestive process.

Keep in mind that water should not be used as a substitute for chewing your food and propelling it into the stomach.

91. Are antibiotic residues in chicken a health problem?

It is a fact that antibiotics are used to maintain the health of animals and subsequently, low residues of antibiotics may be present in some of the food we eat. The 1999-2000 National Residue Survey monitoring program found that in nearly 5000 samples of beef, sheep, pork, chicken and game meat tested, less than 3% had residues of antibiotics, with less than 0.3% having residues above the maximum permissible limit.

There is currently significant community concern in Australia about the presence of antibiotic residue in our food supply and the potential for the development of antibiotic resistance in humans.

Antibiotic resistance in humans is considered to be the result of the overuse of antibiotics. Due to community concern, an expert committee was established to assess the issue and they found it highly unlikely that the consumption of antibiotic residues in food would lead to the development of resistance. This is due to the residue levels already being very low and most likely reduced further by cooking, food processing and digestion.

What is being done about the use of antibiotics in food? Food Standards Australia New Zealand is working with other government agencies to develop strategies that reduce the transfer of bacteria from animals to food. In addition, antibiotic use in food animals is monitored and enforced by the Australian Pesticides and Veterinary Medicines Authority.

92. Is cranberry juice useful against urinary tract infections?

Possibly. For some time cranberry juice has been recommended as a way to prevent or treat urinary tract infections (UTI's). From the limited number of scientific studies conducted to date, it seems that regular drinking of cranberry juice does reduce the recurrence of UTI's in women. A recent Cochrane review of cranberry and urinary tract infection concluded that it is not clear what is the optimum dosage or method of administration (e.g. juice, tablets or capsules). Further properly designed studies with relevant outcomes are needed.

Anyone can get a urinary tract infection but the condition is more prevalent in women than men, the likelihood increases with age and is highest in institutionalised older women.

Until more is known, if you suffer from recurrent UTI's, you may want to try including a small amount of cranberry juice in your daily diet.

93. Does eating before bedtime disturb sleep?

Mealtimes are really an individual preference. Some people may find that it is uncomfortable to eat close to going to bed and this in turn will disturb sleep. Others may not find this to be the case.

In our fast paced world mealtimes seem to have become quite flexible and this is not always in a positive sense. When I was growing up my mum had dinner on the table religiously at 6pm and we all sat down and ate together. This seems to be a thing of the past as we are working longer hours and may have children and other family commitments that prevent us from eating our evening meal at a civilised hour. You may be eating dinner quite late and find that it is getting close to your bedtime.

There is also the question of what you are eating prior to sleeping. Snacking on chocolate, biscuits and cake (which are all high in fat) is not a great choice before you lie down for 8 hours of sleep. The evening is when your body is least active and therefore not burning a lot of fuel.

Essentially, you are the best judge of your own body but if you are experiencing disturbed sleep, acid reflux or other problems, then have a look at your eating habits before bed.

94. Do you need to detox your body regularly?

The human body is very clever. So clever, that it rids itself of toxins whenever they come by, using helpful organs like the lungs, liver, kidneys, also aided by our gastrointestinal tract and our immune system. The liver plays a leading role as most of the end products of digestion of food are transported directly to the liver and poisons and drugs are metabolised and detoxified in the liver. You do not need to externally detox your body and there is no scientific evidence to suggest that detox diets actually work.

Detoxifying the body is not new, but suddenly detox diets are really quite fashionable. Apparently, if you are feeling a bit low and lacking in energy, a spot of detox will do the trick.

There are many 'detox' diets around and all fit into the 'fad diet' category. These diets often remove whole food groups or may rely on liquids only, and if followed for any length of time can actually be quite dangerous. This is especially so for children, teenagers, pregnant or breastfeeding women and the elderly.

If you want to gain energy and get revitalised it is far easier and more effective to reduce your intake of cigarettes, alcohol, saturated and trans fats, sugar and sugary foods. Plus, think about boosting your intake of fruit, vegetables and whole grains and, of course, get your body moving.

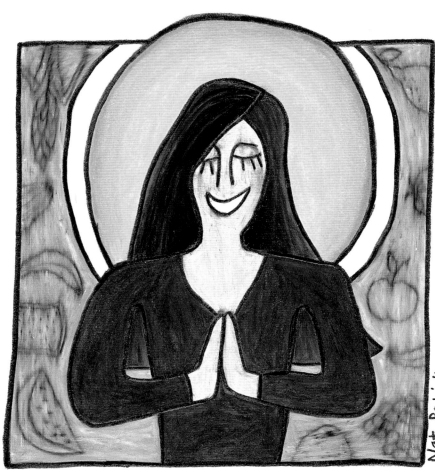

95. I've given up smoking, is weight gain inevitable?

It is possible, if you don't control it. If you quit smoking, weight gain can occur but it is certainly preventable. Interestingly, a study in 2005 found that the most common reason women are reluctant to quit smoking is fear of weight gain! Numerous studies have shown that cigarette smoking does suppress body weight and appetite and quitting smoking is commonly followed by weight gain. One study reported that the average weight gain following smoking cessation is between 2-5 kg. In the short term, nicotine does increase energy expenditure and metabolic rate, which may explain why smokers tend to have a lower body weight than non-smokers and why weight gain often occurs following smoking cessation.

Apart from the obvious drawbacks of smoking such as lung and other cancers, there is an increased risk of diabetes and resulting increased risk of cardiovascular disease.

A group of researchers in 2008 looked at weight gain and smoking cessation rates in women and found that the women who exercised while quitting smoking successfully prevented weight gain.

Quitting smoking improves your health outlook significantly, so there is no point substituting one bad habit for another and eating the wrong foods. Don't pick up high fat snack foods instead of cigarettes. Watch out for the alcohol at parties and social occasions and plan your food intake instead of reaching for the quickest choice, which may not always be the best choice. And remember to exercise and get your metabolism going.

96. Does eating celery burn more calories than the food contains?

Celery is not the easiest food to eat and it certainly does give your jaw a good workout. Two (10cm long) sticks of raw celery contains 20 kilojoules (kJ) of energy, is 95% water and has zero fat with only traces of various vitamins and minerals.

The amount of energy that you expend while eating is roughly 9 kJ per minute, and let's assume that it would take somewhere in the vicinity of 5 minutes to get through those crunchy stalks. This would mean that you are burning up around 43 kJ to eat the celery and it's only providing approximately 20 kJ. However, the figures for energy expenditure while eating are approximations and will depend on the type of food that you are consuming.

So it would seem that yes, you are burning more calories eating the celery than you are gaining from the vegetable itself. Certainly this does not mean you should shun celery, it's heaps better for you than a package of potato chips and offers a satisfying crunch. Make it part of a midday snack with peanut butter, sultanas or almonds and the healthy boost will curb any cravings.

97. Are oysters really an aphrodisiac?

No. Although there is no scientific basis for this theory, perhaps the impotence effect of zinc deficiency is where the secret behind oysters and their aphrodisiac effect lies.

Oysters are by far the richest food source of zinc. Zinc is a mineral that our bodies need for growth and repair and is essential for sexual maturation. One dozen oysters contain close to 79 mg of zinc while the closest non-seafood competitor is liver (100 grams) at 7.6 mg.

Given that our zinc requirements are approximately 12 mg daily, one dozen oysters are not needed every single day! Other sources of zinc include seafood, lean meat and poultry. If a deficiency occurs in children, this can result in growth failure and delay in sexual maturity and in adults, deficiency may result in dermatitis, loss of hair, poor immunity and impotence.

It is interesting to note that zinc deficiency is now included on the World Health Organisation's (WHO) global burden of disease list and one third of the world is at high risk of zinc deficiency.

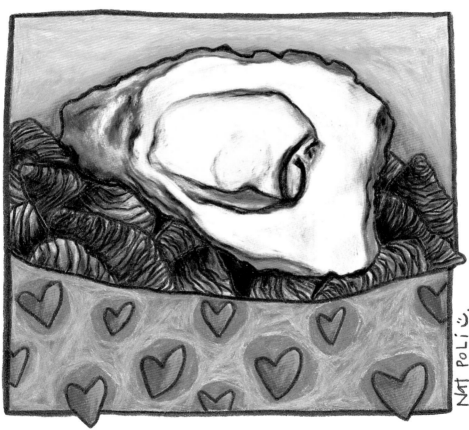

98. Is honey safe for babies to eat?

No. Honey is not recommended for children under 12 months of age due to a risk of contracting a disease known as Infant Botulism. Infant Botulism results from the absorption of a neurotoxin produced by ingested bacteria (Clostridium Botulinum). It is an age-restricted disease as it occurs in babies up to 12 months old due to their immature digestive systems. This disease affects all major racial and ethnic groups and both sexes and has been reported in all European countries, Japan, Australia and Argentina. 90% of cases are reported in the US. It was first identified in 1978.

The symptoms of Infant Botulism are a history of constipation followed by weakness, inability to suck and swallow and may lead to respiratory problems. The syndrome at the severe end of the spectrum can be life threatening. The Clostridium Botulinum organism has been identified in honey, vacuum cleaner dust and soil.

It is reported that contaminated honey is found throughout the world with up to 6-10% of samples containing Clostridium Botulinum spores. Honey is an internationally traded product and therefore Infant Botulism can be expected anywhere.

Given that honey is not an essential food for babies aged 12 months and under, it is best to avoid this food until they are older.

99. Is it healthier to eat three meals per day or lots of smaller meals?

It is your overall food intake that matters, not whether you eat three meals per day or whether you prefer to graze.

Your lifestyle will probably dictate whether you are a three meal per day person or a 'grazer.' The term 'grazing' is so called because cows like to do the same thing. You may not like to think of yourself out in the field chomping down on grass but 'grazing' here means snacking or having 5-6 smaller 'meals' spread out over the day.

Grazing is fine but do keep an eye on what and how much you are actually eating over the day. It can be easy to exceed your daily energy requirements through regular snacking, so make sure that you don't fill up on biscuits, cakes, lollies, chocolate and chips. These types of foods are high in sugar, fat and salt and low in fibre and are certainly not good for your health, but you knew that already!

If you prefer to graze, make sure that you include all of the essential food groups such as fruit and vegetables, cereals and dairy products. Remember to top up on fluids and drink either water or milk and skip the soft drinks.

"The Great enemy of the truth is very often not the lie deliberate, contrived and dishonest, but the myth, persistent, persuasive, and unrealistic. Belief in myths allows the comfort of opinion without the discomfort of thought." - John F Kennedy

About Julie

Julie has over 17 years experience in the public, sports and corporate health and performance industry. To back up this practical experience, Julie is degree qualified in nutrition and health promotion and is an Accredited Practising Dietitian. Julies experience and qualifications enable her to deliver the most current and groundbreaking advice available. She has helped thousands of people achieve personal success through eating well.

How you can work with Julie

Julie is a speaker, coach and author, who works with individuals, teams and businesses to assist them in achieving peak performance.

Email Julie for more information:
julie@juliemeek.com

To receive your FREE special report

"Top tips on raising your energy and productivity."

visit www.juliemeek.com

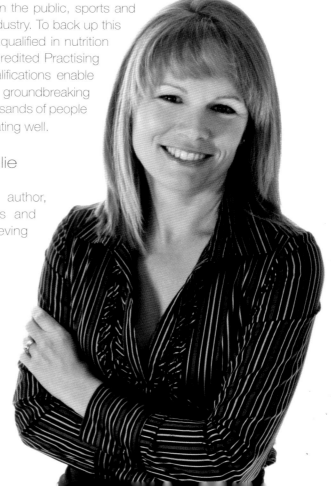

References

Calculations and Nutrient Values (relevant to various Questions)
Wahlqvist M, Briggs D. Food Facts. Melbourne: Penguin Books; 1984.
Mahan LK, Escott-Stump S, editors. Krause's Food and nutrition therapy. 12th ed. St Louis : Elsevier Saunders; 2007.

Question 1
Engler M, Engler M. The emerging role of flavonoid-rich cocoa and chocolate in cardiovascular health and disease. Nutrition Reviews 2006; 64: 109- 119.
Ariefdjohan MW, Savaiano DA. Chocolate and cardiovascular health. Nutrition Reviews 2005; 63: 427– 431.

Question 4
European Journal of Clinical Nutrition 2007; 61: 226-232.

Question 5
Baghurst K. Nutrient Reference Values: insights for weight loss diets. Perspectives, Nutrition News and Views 2007; 23: 4.

Question 6
Australian Institute of Health and Welfare. Australia's Health 2008 [Report];2008.

Question 8
Stanton R. The Art of Sensible Dieting How to Avoid the Weight Loss Rip-offs. Australia: Ellsyd Press; 1986.

Question 9 and 78
Commonwealth Department of Health and Ageing and National Health and Medical Research Council. Food for Health, Dietary Guidelines for Australian Adults. Canberra: Commonwealth Department of Health and Ageing and National Health and Medical Research Council; 2003.

Question 11
Burke V, Giangiulio N, Gillam HF, Beilin LJ et al. Health promotion in couples adapting to a shared lifestyle. Health Education Research 1999; 14: 269-288.
Sobal J, Rauschenbach B, Frongillo E. Marital status changes and body weight changes: A US longitudinal analysis. Social Science and Medicine 2003; 56: 1543.

Question 16
Diamond H, Diamond M. Fit for life. USA: Warner Books; 1985.

Question 23
Dorlands Pocket Medical Dictionary. 30th ed. Philidelphia: Saunders/Elsevier; 2003. Leukonychia; p. 331.

Question 24

Savaiano D, Boushey C, McCabeG. Lactose intolerance symptoms assessed by meta-analysis: a grain of truth that leads to exaggeration. J Nutr 2006; 136: 1107-13.

Montalto M, Curigliano V, Santoro L, Vastola M, Cammarota G, Manna R, et al. Management and treatment of lactose malabsorption. World J Gastroenterol 2006; 12:187-91.

Question 25

Australian and New Zealand Bone Mineral Society. Calcium and Bone Health – Position Statement [homepage on the internet]. c2006 [updated 2008 July 22nd ; cited 2008 August]. Available from www.anzbms.org.au.

Question 28

Mahan LK, Escott-Stump S, editors. Krause's Food and nutrition therapy. 12th ed. St Louis : Elsevier Saunders; 2007.

Questions 31, 69, 72, 81

Food Labelling Laws www.foodstandards.gov.au

Nutrient Information Calculator www.foodstandards.gov.au

Question 42

Egg Nutrition Advisory Group. Eggs and risk of cardiovascular disease – Position Statement [homepage on the internet]. c2008 [updated 2009 Jan ; cited 2008 August]. Available from www.enag.org.au.

Question 53

Burke L, Deakin V, editors. Clinical sports nutrition. 3rd ed. North Ryde: McGraw Hill; 2006.

Cardwell G. Gold medal nutrition. 4th ed. Lower Mitcham: Human Kinetics; 2006.

Question 54

Gatorade Sports Science Institute (Experts on the Science of Protein and Exercise), June 2007.

Question 55

Cardwell G. Gold medal nutrition. 4th ed. Lower Mitcham: Human Kinetics; 2006.

Lemon P. Effect of exercise on dietary protein requirements. Int J of Sports Nutrition. 1998; 8: 426-447.

National Health and Medical Research Council. Recommended Dietary Intakes for use in Australia. Canberra: National Health and Medical Research Council; 1991.

Tarnopolsky M. Clinical sports nutrition. Sydney: McGraw Hill; 2000.

Question 57

Stanton R. Healthy Eating for Australian Families. Millers Point: Millers Books; 2007.

Question 58

Sport Dietitians Australia. Cramps and stitches [Fact Sheet]. South Melbourne: Sports Dietitians Australia; June 2009.

Question 59

Burke L. The complete guide to sports performance. Sydney: Allen and Unwin; 1995.

Sport Dietitians Australia. Sports drinks [Fact Sheet]. South Melbourne: Sports Dietitians Australia; June 2009.

Question 61

Burke LM, Maughan RJ. Alcohol in sports. In: Maughan RJ, ed. IOC Encyclopedia on Sports Nutrition. London: Blackwell, 2000:405-16.

O'Brien C. Alcohol and sport: impact of social drinking on recreational and competitive sports performance. Sports Med 1993; 15: 71-7.

Question 62

Sport Dietitians Australia. Eating and drinking before sport [Fact Sheet]. South Melbourne: Sports Dietitians Australia; April 2009.

Question 64

Burke L, Heeley P. Dietary supplements and nutritional ergogenic aids in sport. In: Burke L, Deakin V, editors. Clinical sports nutrition. 3rd ed. North Ryde: McGraw Hill; 2006.

Question 65

Burke L, Desbrow B, Minehan M. Dietary supplements and nutritional ergogenic aids in sport. In: Burke L, Deakin V, editors. Clinical sports nutrition. 3rd ed. North Ryde: McGraw Hill; 2006.

Question 71

Baghurst P. In: The Role of Red Meat in Healthy Australian Diets. Nutrition and Dietetics 2007; 64: Suppl 4 S173.

Question 76

Ojha R, Amanatidis S, Petocz P, Samman S. Dietitians and Naturopaths require evidence-based nutrition information on organic food. Nutrition and Dietetics 2007; 64: 31-36.

Question 77

Probiotica Volume 11, 2000

Question 79

National Nutrition Survey: Nutrient Intakes and Physical Measurements, Australia 1995

Question 83

Champagne CM. Dietary interventions on blood pressure: the dietary approaches to stop hypertension trials (DASH) trials. Nutrition Reviews 2006; 64: 2.

Fleet JC. DASH without the dash (of salt) can lower blood pressure. Nutrition Reviews 2001; 59(9): 291- 294.

Question 87

Euromonitor International. Vitamins and dietary supplements Report. May 2008. Available at www.euromonitor.com

Question 89 and 91

(Scientific Assessment of the Public Health and Safety of Poultry Meat, Food Standards Australia. Nov 2005)

JETACAR Report: www.health.gov.au/pubhlth/strateg/jetacar

Australian National Residue Survey: www.affa.gov.au/nrs

Food Standards Australia New Zealand. Antibiotics in the Food Supply [pamphlet]. Australia: Food Standards Australia New Zealand; 2001.

Question 92

Kuzminski LN. Cranberry juice and urinary tract infections: is there a beneficial relationship? Nutrition Reviews 1996; 54 (11): S87-90.

Kontiokari T, Nuutinen KM, Pokka T et al. Randomised trial of cranberry-lingonberry juice and Lactobacillus GG drink for the prevention of urinary tract infections in women. British Medical Journal (Int Ed) 2001; 322: 1571-1574.

McMurdo MET, Bissett LY, Price RJG, Phillips G, Crombie IK.. Does ingestion of cranberry juice reduce symptomatic urinary tract infections in older people in hospital? A double-blind, placebo-controlled trial. Age and Ageing 2005; 34: 256.

Jepson RG, Craig JC. Cranberries for reducing urinary tract infections. Cochrane Database System Review 2008; Jan 23 (1):CD001321.

Question 95

Chaney E, Sheriff S. Weight gain among women during smoking cessation: testing the effects of a multi-faceted program. AAOHN Journal. 2008; 56: 99-105.

Question 96

McArdle WD, Katch FI, Katch VL. Sports and exercise nutrition. 3rd ed. USA: Lippincott, Williams and Wilkins; 2008.

Question 98

Kakara, FV, Papazoglou KG, Sideri GI, Papadatos JH. Severe infant botulism with cardiac arrest. Journal of Paediatric Neurology 2007; 5: 175- 178.

Brook I. Infant botulism. Journal of Perinatology 2007; 27 (3): 175- 181.

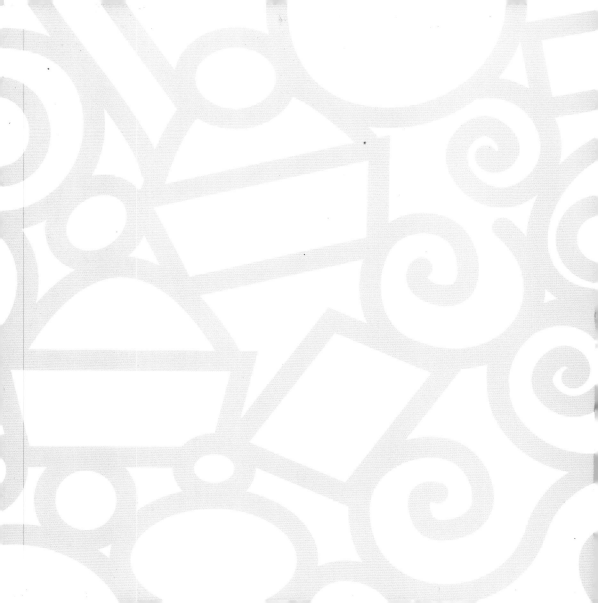